# Oral Placement Therapy for Speech Clarity and Feeding

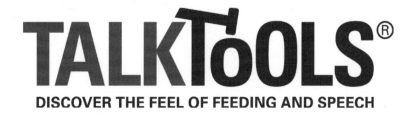

Copyright © 2009 by ITI and Sara Rosenfeld-Johnson
All rights reserved. This book or parts thereof, may not be
reproduced in any form without permission

Research about oral-motor intervention is ongoing and subject to interpretation. Although all reasonable efforts have been made to include the most accurate information in this manual, there can be no guarantee that what we know about this complex subject will not change with time. While the opinions and techniques contained herein are the cumulative effect of the author's efforts, the author, publisher or producer can accept no responsibility for the implementation of the contents of this work. Consumers are advised to consult with experts before beginning any therapy program that includes these techniques.

Library of Congress Cataloging in Publication Date
Rosenfeld-Johnson, Sara, 1948 --
Speech and Language Pathologist M.S., CCC/SLP

Oral Placement Therapy for Speech Clarity and Feeding

I. Title
2001 01 -- 103146
ISBN 1-932460-00-4
(Previous ISBN 1-893660-01-X 3rd ed)

Manufactured in the United States of America

FOURTH EDITION

Cover Photography by Deborah K. O'Brien
Interior Illustrations by Monica Pizarro

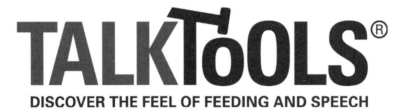

DISCOVER THE FEEL OF FEEDING AND SPEECH

www.talktools.com

**Dedicated**

To my mother, Edythe,
who has always been the "Wind Beneath My Wings"

To my husband, Phil,
who, over the past thirty-five years, has loved me and encouraged
me to become all that I could become

And to our daughters
Rachael, Beth and Lauren,
who are my proudest achievements

# Acknowledgements

## Special thanks go to:

**Lori Overland**, SLP, for her multiple roles in my professional success as:

1. Clinical Supervisor for many years, of Sara R. Johnson, Oral-Motor, Speech Language Associates LLC., in South Salem, New York;

2. CEU Lecturer, on a "Sensory-Motor Approach," for our company, Innovative Therapists International/Talk Tools;

3. A superior SLP to whom I can go when I am at a loss: and

4. A reviewer of the first edition of this manuscript, who added her very professional suggestions

**Diane Bahr**, SLP, for helping me to rewrite this fourth edition for others to truly understand Oral Placement Therapy. Diane is a selfless professional who is always there for me to share an idea or a thought. She is an asset to our profession and refers to herself as, "My sister in speech therapy."

## Additional thanks go to the following people who are well aware of their special place in my professional growth:

Susan Connolly, P.T.
Jennifer Gray, SLP
Renee Roy Hill, SLP
Pamela Marshalla, SLP
June Mathers, Special Educator
Dr. Eleanor Morrison, SLP
Nancy Polow, SLP
Debbie Ripperger
Herbert Rosenfeld
Ilene Rosenfeld
Terry Rosenfeld
Ellie Weinstein, OTR

# Contents

**INTRODUCTION** . . . . . . . . . . . . . . . . . . . . . . . . . . . . . . . . . . . . . . . . . . . . . . . . 1

**INTRODUCTION TO THE FOURTH EDITION** . . . . . . . . . . . . . . . . . . . . . . . . 3

**CHAPTER 1**  STOP!!!!!! . . . . . . . . . . . . . . . . . . . . . . . . . . . . . . . . . . . . . . . . 4

**CHAPTER 2**  HOW TO USE THIS MANUAL EFFECTIVELY . . . . . . . . . . . . . . . 7

**CHAPTER 3**  TARGETING SPEECH SOUNDS . . . . . . . . . . . . . . . . . . . . . . . . .11

SECTION 1 - CONSONANT SOUND PRODUCTION . . . . . . . . . . . . . . . . . . . . . 12
   1. Chart: Placement and Movement Components of Consonant Sound Production 12
   2. Target Phonemes / m, b, p / Suggested Activities . . . . . . . . . . . . . . . . . . 13
   3. Target Phonemes / f, v / Suggested Activities . . . . . . . . . . . . . . . . . . . . . 14
   4. Target Phonemes / θ (th), ð (th) / Suggested Activities . . . . . . . . . . . . . . 15
   5. Target Phonemes / t, d, n, l / Suggested Activities . . . . . . . . . . . . . . . . . . 16
   6. Target Phonemes / k, g / Suggested Activities . . . . . . . . . . . . . . . . . . . . . 17
   7. Target Phonemes / s, z / Suggested Activities . . . . . . . . . . . . . . . . . . . . . 18
   8. Target Phonemes / ʃ(sh), tʃ(ch), ʤ(j) / Suggested Activities . . . . . . . . . . . 19
   9. Target Phonemes / r, vocalic r / Suggested Activities . . . . . . . . . . . . . . . . 20

SECTION 2 - VOWEL SOUND PRODUCTION . . . . . . . . . . . . . . . . . . . . . . . . . 21
   1. Chart: Placement and Movement Components of Vowel Sound Production . . . 22
   2. Target Phonemes / I (ih), i (ee), u (oo), ʊ (oo) / Suggested Activities . . . . . . . . 23
   3. Target Phonemes / ʌ (uh), O, ə (uh), ɔ (aw),  ε (eh) / Suggested Activities . . . . 24
   4. Target Phonemes / æ (a), a (ah) / Suggested Activities . . . . . . . . . . . . . . . 25

**CHAPTER 4**  PHONATION ACTIVITIES . . . . . . . . . . . . . . . . . . . . . . . . . . . . 26
   1. Bubble Blowing Hierachy . . . . . . . . . . . . . . . . . . . . . . . . . . . . . . . . . . 28
   2. "Ah" in Supine . . . . . . . . . . . . . . . . . . . . . . . . . . . . . . . . . . . . . . . . . . 34
   3. Candle Blowing . . . . . . . . . . . . . . . . . . . . . . . . . . . . . . . . . . . . . . . . . 37
   4. Horn Blowing Hierachy . . . . . . . . . . . . . . . . . . . . . . . . . . . . . . . . . . . . 45
   5. Golf Ball Air Hockey . . . . . . . . . . . . . . . . . . . . . . . . . . . . . . . . . . . . . . 51
   6. Echo Horn . . . . . . . . . . . . . . . . . . . . . . . . . . . . . . . . . . . . . . . . . . . . . 54
   7. Microphone . . . . . . . . . . . . . . . . . . . . . . . . . . . . . . . . . . . . . . . . . . . . 56
   8. Kazoo . . . . . . . . . . . . . . . . . . . . . . . . . . . . . . . . . . . . . . . . . . . . . . . . 58

**CHAPTER 5**  RESONATION ACTIVITIES . . . . . . . . . . . . . . . . . . . . . . . . . . 61
   1. Humming #1 . . . . . . . . . . . . . . . . . . . . . . . . . . . . . . . . . . . . . . . . . . . 63
   2. Nose Flute . . . . . . . . . . . . . . . . . . . . . . . . . . . . . . . . . . . . . . . . . . . . . 65
   3. Oral-Nasal Contrasts . . . . . . . . . . . . . . . . . . . . . . . . . . . . . . . . . . . . . 69
   4. Singing-Humming . . . . . . . . . . . . . . . . . . . . . . . . . . . . . . . . . . . . . . . 74

**CHAPTER 6**  ARTICULATION ACTIVITIES . . . . . . . . . . . . . . . . . . . . . . . . . 76

v

SECTION 1 - JAW ACTIVITIES . . . . . . . . . . . . . . . . . . . . . . . . . . . . . . . . . 78

   1. Jaw Grading Bite Blocks . . . . . . . . . . . . . . . . . . . . . . . . . . . . . . . . . . 80

       Natural Bite . . . . . . . . . . . . . . . . . . . . . . . . . . . . . . . . . . . . . . . . . . 80

   2. Jaw Grading Bite Block Exercises . . . . . . . . . . . . . . . . . . . . . . . . . . . 85

   3. Assessment Procedure (Diagnostic) . . . . . . . . . . . . . . . . . . . . . . . . . 89

       Exercise A-Bite Block . . . . . . . . . . . . . . . . . . . . . . . . . . . . . . . . . . 91

       Exercise B-Twin Bite Blocks for Symmetrical Jaw Stability . . . . . . . . . . . 93

       Exercise C Bite Block for Jaw Stability . . . . . . . . . . . . . . . . . . . . . . . . 95

       How to Evaluate Jaw Stability . . . . . . . . . . . . . . . . . . . . . . . . . . . . . 98

       Using the Correct Diagnostic Term . . . . . . . . . . . . . . . . . . . . . . . . . . 99

       Treatment - Therapeutic Technique . . . . . . . . . . . . . . . . . . . . . . . . . 102

   4. Gum Chewing . . . . . . . . . . . . . . . . . . . . . . . . . . . . . . . . . . . . . . . . 108

SECTION 2 - LIP ACTIVITIES . . . . . . . . . . . . . . . . . . . . . . . . . . . . . . . . . 115

   1. Crumbs . . . . . . . . . . . . . . . . . . . . . . . . . . . . . . . . . . . . . . . . . . . . 116

   2. Single-Sip Cup Drinking . . . . . . . . . . . . . . . . . . . . . . . . . . . . . . . . . 119

   3. Kisses . . . . . . . . . . . . . . . . . . . . . . . . . . . . . . . . . . . . . . . . . . . . 122

   4. Humming #2 . . . . . . . . . . . . . . . . . . . . . . . . . . . . . . . . . . . . . . . . 126

   5. Sponge Balsa-Tongue Depressor . . . . . . . . . . . . . . . . . . . . . . . . . . 128

   6. Tongue Depressor for Lip Closure . . . . . . . . . . . . . . . . . . . . . . . . . . 131

   7. Fine Motor Tasks with Lip Closure . . . . . . . . . . . . . . . . . . . . . . . . . . 135

   8. Straw Drinking Hierarchy . . . . . . . . . . . . . . . . . . . . . . . . . . . . . . . . 138

   9. Straw Hierarchy for Thin Liquids . . . . . . . . . . . . . . . . . . . . . . . . . . . 139

  10. Straw Hierarchy for Thickened Liquids . . . . . . . . . . . . . . . . . . . . . . . 145

  11. OO-EE (OO-EE-AH) . . . . . . . . . . . . . . . . . . . . . . . . . . . . . . . . . . . 150

  12. Button Pull . . . . . . . . . . . . . . . . . . . . . . . . . . . . . . . . . . . . . . . . . 152

  13. Cheerio for Lower-Lip Retraction . . . . . . . . . . . . . . . . . . . . . . . . . . . 155

SECTION 3 - TONGUE ACTIVITIES . . . . . . . . . . . . . . . . . . . . . . . . . . . . . 159

   1. Resistance for Tongue Blade Protrusion Production Criteria for / θ (th) ð (th) /. 160

   2. Tongue Blade Retraction - Summary . . . . . . . . . . . . . . . . . . . . . . . . . 164

   3. Tongue Blade Retraction with Resistance . . . . . . . . . . . . . . . . . . . . . . 165

   4. Tongue-Tip Lateralization . . . . . . . . . . . . . . . . . . . . . . . . . . . . . . . . 167

   5. Tongue-Tip Pointing . . . . . . . . . . . . . . . . . . . . . . . . . . . . . . . . . . . 175

   6. Cheerio for Tongue-Tip Elevation . . . . . . . . . . . . . . . . . . . . . . . . . . . 176

   7. Cheerio for Tongue-Tip Depression . . . . . . . . . . . . . . . . . . . . . . . . . 181

   8. Tongue-Tip Up and Down . . . . . . . . . . . . . . . . . . . . . . . . . . . . . . . . 185

   9. Back of Tongue Side Spread - Summary . . . . . . . . . . . . . . . . . . . . . . 190

  10. "EE" . . . . . . . . . . . . . . . . . . . . . . . . . . . . . . . . . . . . . . . . . . . . . . 191

  11. Dinosaur for /r/ Production Criteria for /r/ and the Vocalic /r/ . . . . . . . . . . 197

**SAMPLE PROGRAM PLAN COMPONENTS** . . . . . . . . . . . . . . . . . . . . . . 204

**GLOSSARY** . . . . . . . . . . . . . . . . . . . . . . . . . . . . . . . . 207

**REFERENCES** . . . . . . . . . . . . . . . . . . . . . . . . . . . . . . . . 215

# INTRODUCTION

Thirty-six years ago when I graduated from Teachers College of Columbia University with a Master's of Science Degree in Speech Pathology, I started my professional career with very high hopes. I had been well educated, both at Teachers College, Columbia University, and at Ithaca College, and had confidence in my abilities. By the end of my first year as a public school speech-language pathologist, I was ready to quit the field. I am by nature a perfectionist.

During that first year, each of my 74 "special education" clients made significant gains in language understanding and language usage. Many of them had increased their sentence length by three to four words. Unfortunately, too many of them were more difficult to understand at the end of the year than at the beginning of the year. Their motor systems were unable to support the increased demand being placed on them. Fortunately for me, I did not quit. Instead, I tried to access information from my graduate school professors, professional journals, and anyone who would listen to me.

A few years later I met the two people who would change the way I would look at speech therapy forever. Surprisingly, they were not speech pathologists. Ellie Weinstein, an occupational therapist, and Susan Connelly, a physical therapist, opened my eyes to the necessity of improving muscle function and movement to aid in improving speech and feeding. I will forever be in their debt.

The therapeutic activities presented in this book represent thirty-six years of "figuring out" how to improve speech clarity and feeding skills. Paying attention to oral structural placement and movement systems, while simultaneously increasing utterance length, has been the key to my clients' articulatory successes. I call this Oral Placement Therapy (OPT) and use it as part of both feeding and speech treatment. Over the past 25 years, I expanded my use of OPT to clients of many ages and ability levels. I have incorporated OPT into my program plans for many types of speech disorders (e.g., dysarthria, apraxia of speech voice disorders, fluency disorders and post CVA clients, as well as clients with mild-to-profound levels of hearing loss).

**OPT therapy for speech teaches oral structural placement to clients who cannot produce or imitate speech sounds using traditional auditory or visual input. For these clients, it is critical to expand speech sound production from phonemes and other similar oral movements the client can already produce. Once a client can produce a targeted speech sound using traditional auditory or visual input, speech therapy can progress in a more typical manner. OPT is only a small part of a comprehensive speech and language program and should not be done in isolation. The activities are carefully selected to stimulate the same movements used in the targeted speech production. They can be completed in under 15 minutes and can be used to refocus attention and concentration from a sensory processing perspective.**

Many of the clients who require these techniques have often received traditional auditory and visually based speech facilitation for a number of years, with minimal success. Traditional speech facilitation has not been effective with these clients because there may be a movement or placement disorder. So, before you introduce any of the techniques in this book, you should thoroughly assess the client's motor functioning for speech and feeding. Explain to the parent(s), caregiver(s) and/or the client that no one is at fault for the client's difficulty in learning to produce target speech sounds. Nor is it the fault of the previous speech-language pathologist. You are going to incorporate a new method of oral placement therapy along with the traditional methods for improved results.

OPT is an important addition to traditional speech treatment methods for clients with placement and movement deficits. **It is a tactile-proprioceptive teaching technique which accompanies traditional therapy.** Traditional therapy is primarily auditory and visual. Clients with motor and/or sensory impairments benefit from tactile and proprioceptive components because speech is a tactile-proprioceptive act. OPT is used to improve articulator awareness, placement (dissociation, grading, and direction of movement), stability, and muscle memory; all of these are necessary for the development of speech clarity.

Please remember, the therapies in this book do not replace anything you are currently using. They are the "pieces of the pie or puzzle" that may not have been supplied in our formal education. So do not throw away anything you do now that is working. Try OPT with a few of your most "challenging" speech clients (i.e., those not responding to auditory and visual cueing alone). See how it goes. I hope you have as much success with your clients as I have had with mine.

# INTRODUCTION TO THE FOURTH EDITION
## (and the reason for the name change)

Eight years ago, after I wrote the first edition of *Oral-Motor Exercises for Speech Clarity*, I felt "Now I can relax." I have it all down on paper so other therapists will be able to use my approach to improve their client's speech clarity and feeding skills. How naive I was. I had forgotten why I love being a speech and language pathologist: my client's needs are ever-changing, and the challenge of developing innovative therapies to address their needs is my passion.

The activities in this book have remained the same, but I have made slight changes to many of the chapters as a result of my improved skills as an SLP and the many misunderstandings about what I do.

I am a person who teaches through example, so let me use that same method to explain the name change of this book. You go out to a restaurant, and the server comes to your table and asks you if you want dessert. If you answer "yes" to that question the server still does not know what you want. The word dessert describes a category of choices not the specific choice. For many years the term "oral-motor therapy" has been used in that same way -- as an umbrella term. Misunderstandings about what I teach have been used to tell therapists not to use this very effective therapy. It is for this reason I have decided to take my friends' (Nancy Kaufman, SLP, and Diane Bahr, SLP) suggestions. I am indebted to both women for their continual support of my work.

The work I do is based upon the premise that some clients cannot achieve the appropriate placement or movement patterns associated with speech clarity and feeding skill development when they are asked to imitate the modeled production. For these clients an additional cueing system is needed: tactile. Oral Placement Therapy (OPT) is used for clients who need a tactile cue to teach articulator placements needed for speech. Only speech movements are targeted in this therapy.

In closing, I would like to thank the over 12,000 therapists, special educators and parents who have purchased a copy of one of the earlier editions of this book. I continue to value your support of my work and look forward to hearing all of your success stories. Please feel free to contact me or one of my associates with comments or questions at www.talktools.com.

Sara Rosenfeld-Johnson MS, CCC-SLP
Speech-Language Pathologist

# CHAPTER 1
## STOP !!!!!!!!!!!!!!!!!!!!!!!!!!!!!!!!!!!!!!!!!!!!

Before you try any of the activities in this manual, it is important to understand why we use certain techniques with certain clients. Your tendency may be to initially skip through this section, but I hope you will STOP and read about what is critical to the success of any oral placement intervention. Although this is a step-by-step technique for improving speech clarity and feeding skills, it is not a "cookbook." The word "cookbook" implies that all you need to do is follow the instructions and you will succeed. The problem with that idea is when working with our clients, no two people are the same. If you treat them the same, you will miss key elements to their success. So, follow me through this book for a better understanding behind the reasons for using oral placement techniques as a part of your speech therapy interventions. Remember, this therapy is never done in isolation and must be connected to feeding and/or speech movements.

**The basic premise of this book is that standard speech utilizes normal muscle movement.** Each chapter is designed to address a specific placement and motor movement, with the goal of improving speech clarity. Along the way you will also reduce or eliminate maladaptive oral habits such as drooling. For those of you who work with clients who do not have oral placement or motor-planning deficits, these techniques and activities can be beneficial to teach placement cues for your speech clients. Speech is the end result of four critical elements of muscle movement: (1) Awareness of the oral structures, (2) Placement of the oral structures, (3) Stability, endurance, and muscle memory, and (4) Production.

**1. AWARENESS:** Awareness is the sensory component of movement. Remember that movement is based upon sensation. If I were to put a piece of food in your mouth, why would you chew it, because you knew I had placed the food in your mouth, or because you "felt" it? Obviously, it is because you "felt" it. Speech is based upon kinesthetic and proprioceptive feedback (Bahr, 2001; Clark & Ostry, 2005; Fisher, et al., 1991; Schmidt, 1988; Morris & Klein, 1987) and Metalinguistic (Klein, et al., 1991; Koegel, et al., 1986). If a client is unable to "feel" the position of a muscle or has a negative reaction to this "feel," speech clarity will be compromised. It is important to address the client's sensory system as a component of their oral-motor intervention.

Many of you are able to diagnose and treat each of the following sensory categories. If you are new to this type of intervention, it will be critical that you consult with someone trained in sensory integration and processing. Over the years, I have learned a tremendous amount from occupational therapists and physical therapists who are trained in Neuro-Developmental Technique (NDT), Sensory Integration, and fine and gross motor development and pathology.

    **a. Tactile Hypersensitivity/Responsivity:** An overreaction to tactile input.

    <u>Example:</u>    When you approach the client or are about to touch the client there is no obvious reaction. As soon as you touch the client, there is a negative reaction. In a feeding environment, these are the clients who have very specific food preferences and are careful about what they put in their mouths.

    <u>Population:</u>    Tactile hypersensitivity is common in clients with the diagnosis of Cerebral Palsy, ADHD, Autism Spectrum Disorders, various syndromes, visual impairments and other disorders characterized by hypertonia.

b. **Tactile Hyposensitivity/Responsivity:** An underreaction to tactile input.

> Example: These clients seek touch. In a feeding environment, these are the clients who may drool, "food stuff," mouth objects and hands, or have reduced reaction to touch. They may enjoy highly-flavored and crunchy foods.
>
> Population: Tactile hyposensitivity is common in clients with the diagnosis of Down syndrome, Benign Hypotonia and other disorders characterized by hypotonia.

c. **Mixed Tactile Sensitivity/Responsivity:** A combination of hypersensitivity and/or hyposensitivity and/or normal sensitivity.

> Example: In order to diagnose this type of sensory system, you will have to do a thorough oral assessment. These clients may have "pockets" of sensitivity. Their feeding patterns may be confusing. Reactions to types of input or foods may be inconsistent and contradictory,
>
> Population: Mixed Tactile Sensitivity is common in clients with the diagnosis of Cerebral Palsy, and Sensory Integration Deficits and is commonly seen in clients with the diagnosis of Apraxia.

d. **Fluctuating Tactile Sensitivity/Responsivity:** Responses that change over time.

> Example: In this group of clients, the sensory system can change from day to day or from minute to minute, depending on the amount of stimuli they are receiving. Many of these clients are also diagnosed with Sensory Integration Deficits or Sensory Processing Disorders.
>
> Population: Fluctuating Tactile Sensitivity is common in clients with the diagnosis of Autism, Asperger's Syndrome and PDD.

e. **Tactile Defensiveness/Responsivity:** A tendency to respond negatively or emotionally to tactile input.

> Example: In contrast to the first four sensory diagnoses, this type of sensory reaction is learned. It can, therefore, be superimposed on any of the above sensory systems. The difference is when a client is tactilely defensive, the sensory reaction is anticipated and avoided. There is a lack of "trust" that must be addressed prior to assessing and targeting the actual sensory system.
>
> Population: Tactile Defensiveness is seen in clients with any of the above-described sensory systems.

**2. PLACEMENT:** Therapy tools are used to help the client achieve placement of the articulators. For example, if I want to teach you to close your lips to make the sound of / m /, / b / or / p /, I can do any of the following: (1) Say "Close your lips" (auditory stimuli), (2) Show you my closed lips and instruct you to do what I am doing (visual stimuli), or (3) Place a tongue depressor or a flat-mouthed horn between your lips (tactile stimuli). The last is the OPT technique. Each of the activities in this book uses a "tool" to teach placement (tactile stimuli). Traditionally, once the client has been able to achieve the placement, we jump to production of the targeted speech sound. As a result, we have achieved success with some clients and failed with others. This book addresses those failures. There is a critical step between placement and speech sound production: adequate strength, muscle memory, stability, and endurance.

For clients with the diagnosis of apraxia and childhood apraxia of speech (CAS), placement activities and tactile cues are the keys to improved speech clarity and feeding skills. Tactile cues are given, in addition to visual and auditory cues, to assist in teaching motor planning for speech sound production. Because tactile learning provides the foundation for motor movement, tactile cues to supplement traditional speech therapy (auditory and visual cueing) help clients improve skill levels through maximizing all sensory systems.

**3. STABILITY/ENDURANCE/MUSCLE MEMORY:** Whereas therapy "tools" are used to achieve placement, repetitions are used to increase stability and endurance and/or to change/ develop **muscle memory**. Let's assume you have taught a client to say / m /, while holding the tongue depressor between his or her lips. What would happen when you remove the tongue depressor? Would the client transition that "placement" technique to production of the / m / in a word? In some cases, yes. In many cases, no. One possible reason for the failure may be that the muscles do not have the muscle memory, stability and endurance to support the placement of / m / within a word. Another possibility may be that habit is interfering with the transition. The client is used to saying b/m. The third possibility is that adequate strength and habit are interfering with carryover of the movement into speech sound production. In any of these scenarios, repetition of the placement exercise will be necessary.

Each technique and activity in the book is divided into "Steps." Once placement is taught in a specific "Step," the number of repetitions needed to meet the "Criteria for Success" will be given. The number of repetitions is based upon stability, endurance, adequate strength, and muscle memory requirements and must be followed closely if success is expected. If you are having trouble getting a client to cooperate for the necessary number of repetitions, for example in the Horn Blowing Hierarchy, please don't go to the next horn on the hierarchy. Instead, step back and brainstorm how you can motivate the client to achieve the required number of repetitions before going on.

**4. PRODUCTION:** Patience is a virtue. If you can keep yourself from working on production during continuous speech until after you have achieved the "Criteria for Success" for Placement, carryover of the speech sound into conversational speech will be easy. The problem here is that so many of us have been taught to work on production of the speech sound during the initial session. In our clinic, the hardest thing for our new therapists to do is wait until the "Criteria for Success" for Placement has been met. Keep reminding yourself that standard speech is superimposed on normal muscle movement. If you teach the client to say the sound prematurely, you may get a distortion with compensatory strategies being used or standard production in isolation, but the weak oral musculature or the engrained habit pattern may inhibit the client's ability to use the sound functionally at the conversational level. When the "Criteria for Success" for a single speech sound or group of speech sounds is identified, those phonemes will be targeted at the beginning of each specific activity.

Remember, that each session must include direct work on speech and language using the skills the client has already mastered with traditional speech therapy techniques or OPT interventions.

# CHAPTER 2
# HOW TO USE THIS MANUAL MOST EFFECTIVELY

The techniques and activities are divided into articulator groups. Let's begin by thinking about speech from a slightly different angle. Try to envision speech as air that is changed and directed by a hierarchy of muscle and articulatory movements. The air that is not used for speech movements is known as air for (**1**) **Respiration.** After inhalation, the grading of the abdominal muscles results in controlled exhalation of the airflow. The controlled outward airflow (grading) is used for (**2**) **Phonation.** The air then moves into the oral cavity and is shaped by the position of the oral structures and the functioning of the velum for (**3**) **Resonation.** This same air is then directed through the nose or through the mouth. There it is shaped by the muscles and structures of (**4**) **Articulation:** the jaw, lips and tongue. **Dissociation** and **grading** in each muscle group is necessary for standard co-articulation. In other words, the jaw must move independently from the lips and the tongue (dissociation). If the jaw is used to move either or both of these articulators, speech clarity will be compromised.

So, where do you start? Your first goal will be to establish a stable seating posture. Neuro-Developmental Technique (NDT) teaches us that stability in the body is a necessary component of mobility in the mouth. If you have been trained in NDT or other gross motor training, establishing a stable posture will be within your abilities. If, however, you do not have this or similar training, it will be critical that you consult with a trained SLP, an occupational therapist or a physical therapist, who can assist you in establishing appropriate body support for this first step toward improving speech clarity. Constant attention to maintaining the stable posture, once it has been identified, will be a challenge as well as a requirement.

For many clients, the optimal position will be in a chair or other support structure which supports a 90-degree angle in the pelvis, knees and ankles. Both feet should be supported on the floor or on a flat surface. I use either Dysum or Rubbermaid Shelf Liner (the puffy type), cut to fit the chair surface or the floor surface to inhibit sliding out of stability. Other clients will achieve maximum stability using a wedge, a therapy ball, a bolster, a prone stander or a therapeutic chair. Remember that each client is unique; therefore, attention to their specific stability needs will be your first responsibility. Maintaining a stable posture throughout the Oral Placement for Feeding and Speech components of each session, will be a requirement for assessment as well as therapeutic intervention. Homework assignments should also be practiced in a stable posture to ensure maximum success.

During your assessment, it will be necessary to evaluate the skills in each articulator group. If a deficit is identified in the structures of phonation, you must begin there while continuing to address speech sound production. If motor functioning for phonation is intact, but motor functioning for resonation is weak, you must begin with resonation while continuing to address speech sound production. If the motor functioning for phonation and resonation are intact, you will target articulation. The muscles and structures for articulation also follow a hierarchy. See the picture at right. Pretend you are at a circus watching acrobats perform. Look at the Ball on the top of the pyramid. Imagine that this

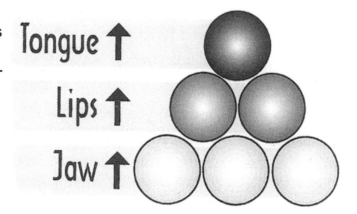

is the best acrobat in the world. Now tell me what would happen if the three Balls (acrobats) on the bottom were weak or unstable? That's right the acrobats at the top would fall off. Transition this idea to the muscles and structures of articulation. The three acrobats on the bottom represent the jaw. The two acrobats in the middle represent the lips. The single acrobat on the top represents the tongue. This picture describes the hierarchy of function known as **dissociation**.

Therefore, if you have identified instability in the jaw, lips and tongue, you would begin with jaw activities. If the jaw is stable but there is instability in placement and movement of the lips and tongue, you would begin with lip activities. If the jaw and lips are stable and can move independently (dissociated), then you would begin with tongue activities. **If there are deficits in the jaw, lips and tongue, you will begin at the highest level before failure in each of the activities in the chapter entitled, "Articulation."**

1. **Respiration:** Air for respiration is equal in amount and duration, as it pertains to inhalation and exhalation.

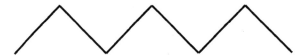

2. **Phonation:** Air that is used for speech is unique. The amount is the same, but the inhalation is quick and the exhalation is prolonged or controlled.

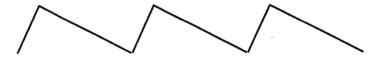

If the client is unable to prolong oral airflow sufficiently during speech production, intelligibility will be reduced. Many of these clients will develop compensatory patterns to extend their statement length. Here are some compensatory possibilities which might be observed. The client will:

1. speak in shorter phrases than his/her linguistic skill levels would support.
2. use compensatory body postures to "push out" more air.
3. speak on inhalation.
4. speak on a combination of inhalation and exhalation (supplemental air).

The activities outlines in the chapter titled, "**Phonation**," will address the inability to sufficiently control oral airflow. Abdominal muscle grading will be the target. Please realize, however, that each of the activities in this book deals with a variety of placement and movement deficits. Your reason for using a specific activity, for example, "**Horn Blowing Hierarchy**," may be to improve abdominal grading. Do note, however, that this same hierarchy addresses improved functioning of the velum, jaw, lips and tongue as a part of standard speech sound production.

Once adequate abdominal support is either identified or established through intervention you will begin the activities in the chapter titled, "**Resonation.**" There will be certain criteria, which must be met, before you introduce the activities and techniques in this chapter. The criteria are noted in the Suggestion Section of each activity.

Activities in the chapter titled, "**Articulation**," are presented in a hierarchy.

**A.  Jaw Activities:**  The jaw activities are first.  If jaw instability has been identified, you must address this deficit before you can work on establishing dissociation of lips from jaw or tongue from jaw.  Jaw activities address:  jaw control, jaw symmetry, jaw alignment, jaw stability, jaw grading and cheek muscle control as movement patterns directly associated with feeding and speech production.

**B.  Lip Activities:**  The lip activities are next. When we observe normal development, we note that functional lip dissociation develops in a hierarchy:

    **1.)**    **Close**
            **Open**

    **2.)**    **Protrusion/Rounding**
            **Retraction**

    **3.)**    **Lower Lip Retraction**
            **Lower Lip Protrusion**

Remember that in order to continue to work on any activity in this chapter the jaw must remain stable during practice.  If the jaw cannot remain stable, despite numerous attempts to achieve stability, you will have to go back to the jaw activities, continue jaw activities simultaneously, or provide external jaw support.  Note that some activities in this chapter require prerequisite jaw skills.

**C.  Tongue Activities:**  The tongue activities are next.  When we observe normal development, we note that functional tongue dissociation also develops in a hierarchy.  We should not expect our clients to perform a higher level of function than their developmental skills allow.  For example, if your targeted speech sound(s) require dissociated tongue-tip elevation and your client is still using excessive tongue protrusion during function, you will have to go back to level 2 activities, "**Tongue Retraction**."  Once you have taught adequate retraction skills, you will then be able to go on to "**Tongue Lateralization**" activities and finally on to "**Tongue-Tip Elevation**" activities. Note that some activities in this chapter require prerequisite jaw and lip skills.

    **1.) Retraction - Protraction:** Equal range of motion (balance)

    Function for feeding:  Suckle for breast or bottle feeding

    **2.) Retraction** (increases and becomes more prominent movement)
    **Protraction** (reduces)

    *Function for feeding:*  Cup Drinking, Spoon Feeding, Straw Drinking
    *Function for speech:*  This placement is needed for all sounds in English with the exception of the voiced and voiceless "th."

**3.) Retraction (stability)** - Lateralization of tip

**a.) Midline to both sides:**

*Function for feeding:* Move bolus from midline to the back molar(s) for safe/effective chewing
*Function for speech:* This placement is not used for speech sound production but is a prerequisite skill for tongue-tip elevation and depression which is needed for speech
**Note:** Remember true lateralization is achieved inside of the mouth, with retraction most prominent, for stability. Once the back of the tongue is stabilized on the palate, the tongue-tip can move independently to touch the lower back molars on alternating sides of the mouth. When you attempt to assess tongue lateralization outside of the mouth, realize that you are testing tongue "wagging" which has nothing to do with speech clarity and is a waste of time; it is not true tongue lateralization. The tongue must remain in the oral cavity as it is for speech.

**b.) Across Midline:**

*Function for feeding:* Move bolus from the back molar(s) on one side of the mouth to the back molar(s) on the other side of the mouth for safe/effective chewing
*Function for speech:* This placement is not used for speech sound production but is a prerequisite skill for tongue-tip elevation and depression which is needed for speech.
**Note:** This movement pattern is the criteria for teaching independent self-feeding of cubed solids.

**4.) Retraction (Stability)** - Tongue-Tip Elevation/Depression

*Function for feeding:* Manipulate the bolus and stabilize the tongue for swallowing
*Function for speech:* Produce tongue-tip elevation and tongue-tip depression speech sounds: "t, d, n, l, s, z, sh, ch, j, k, g"

**5.) Retraction (Stability)** - Back of Tongue Side Spread

*Function for speech:* Produce back of tongue side spread phonemes and all speech sounds in a co-articulated manner as a result of stability at the back of the tongue which allows for mobility of the blade and tip. Without this skill, speech clarity at the conversational level will be compromised.

**Note:** The words presented in bold are defined in the Glossary as they are used in this book.

# C H A P T E R  3
# TARGETING SPEECH SOUNDS
## Choosing The Right Activities For Your Client's Specific Needs

Any basic articulation test can be used to describe a client's oral phoneme-error pattern or how a client sounds when he/she says a specific speech sound. These tests do not, however, give you oral placement or movement information, unless you watch how the client says the sounds as the test is being administered. In order to develop a Program Plan utilizing both traditional and OPT techniques, you will have to know how the client's articulators are positioned during the production of each speech sound, in addition to the phonetic description of that speech sound. An **OPT Articulation Form** can be used to chart both the acoustic and articulator placement information you receive as you watch and listen to your client's performance on any standardized articulation test.

## CONSONANT SOUND PRODUCTION

The following chart and subsequent pages outline the standard oral placement and movement components of each consonant in the areas of: Jaw Height, Tongue Placement, Lip Placement, Voicing and Resonance. After reviewing the information on the next page, it will be beneficial to compare the listed characteristics with the information you charted on the client's OPT Articulation Form. In this way you will be able to see any placement deficits. For example, if the client uses an interdental production of /p/ consistently on the standardized articulation test you can use that information to identify the following placement deficits:

| **Characteristics for standard production of /p/** | **Client's interdental production of /p/** |
|---|---|
| **High Jaw Placement** - Yes | **High Jaw Placement** - No |
| **Lip Closure** - Yes | **Lip Closure** - No |
| **Tongue Retraction** - Yes | **Tongue Retraction** - No |

In this example, the client did not use a developmental substitution but instead used a pattern of articulator distortion. Once you see this evidence on paper you can see the muscle placements which need to be addressed for this client to produce the standard /p/: high jaw placement with lip closure and tongue retraction. The standard oral placement and movement components of vowel sound production can be found in the chart on page 12. When you identify which articulators are being used incorrectly, you will be able to choose **The Right Activities For Your Client's Specific Needs.**

Since not all placement and movement components of speech sound production can be seen, let me make a suggestion: Choose one phoneme. Say the sound as you say it (i.e., the standard way). Use kinesthetic and priopriceptive feedback to "feel" within your mouth where your articulators are placed. Compare your articulator placement with the placement described in the chart on the next page for that specific speech sound. Now, say the sound as your client just said it, using their error production. Use kinesthetic and priopriceptive feedback to "feel" what you had to do orally to make their error sound production. Which articulators did you move? Once you determine which component of standard production your client is using incorrectly, you will know **The Right Activities For Your Client's Specific Needs.**

# PLACEMENT AND MOVEMENT Components of Consonant Sounds

| Phoneme | Jaw Height | Tongue Position | Lips | Voicing | Resonance |
|---------|-----------|-----------------|------|---------|-----------|
| m | High | Retracted | Closed | Yes | Nasal |
| r | High | Retracted Back of Tongue: Side Spread | Lower Lip Protrusion/Tension | Yes | Oral |
| vocalic /r/ | High or Medium | Retracted Back of Tongue: Side Spread | Lower Lip Protrusion/Tension | Yes | Oral |
| t | Medium | Retracted Tongue-Tip Elevation | Open | No | Oral |
| ℓ | Medium | Retracted Tongue-Tip Elevation | Open | Yes | Oral |
| s | High | Retracted, Tongue-Tip Elevation or Depression | Open | No | Oral |
| n | High | Retracted Tongue-Tip Elevation | Open | Yes | Nasal |
| z | High | Retracted, Tongue-Tip Elevation or Depression | Open | Yes | Oral |
| ʃ(sh) | High | Retracted Back of Tongue: Side Spread | Rounded | No | Oral |
| b | High | Retracted | Closed | Yes | Oral |
| k | Low | Retracted Tongue-Tip Depression | Open | No | Oral |
| f | High | Retracted | Lower Lip Retracted | No | Oral |
| d | Medium | Retracted Tongue-Tip Elevation | Open | Yes | Oral |
| g | Low | Retracted Tongue-Tip Depression | Open | Yes | Oral |
| tʃ(ch) | High | Retracted, Tongue-Tip Elevation to Back of Tongue: Side Spread | Rounded | No | Oral |
| dʒ(j) | High | Retracted, Tongue-Tip Elevation to Back of Tongue: Side Spread | Rounded | Yes | Oral |
| ð (th) | Medium | Protruded | Open | Yes | Oral |
| θ (th) | Medium | Protruded | Open | No | Oral |
| p | High | Retracted | Closed | No | Oral |
| v | High | Retracted | Lower Lip Retracted | Yes | Oral |
| ŋ(ng) | Low | Retracted Back of Tongue: Side Spread | Open | Yes | Nasal |

# TARGET PHONEMES - / m, b, p /

**Oral Placement Components**

| | |
|---|---|
| **Jaw Height:** | High |
| **Tongue Position:** | Retracted |
| **Lips:** | Closed |

**Suggested Activities:**

**Note:** The following techniques will improve placement and movement skills for the production of / m, b, p /. Not every client will need to use all of the activities. Some activities may be eliminated because the client already demonstrates the "Criteria for Success." A typical therapy session of 30 to 45 minutes will include five activities in addition to traditional speech therapy techniques.

1. Establishing a Natural Bite
2. Bite Block (Jaw Height Level #2)
3. Twin Bite Blocks for Symmetrical Jaw Stability (Jaw Height Level #2)
4. Bite Block for Jaw Stability (Jaw Height Level #2)
5. Gum Chewing
6. Bubble Blowing
7. Horn Blowing
8. Straw Drinking
9. Humming
10. Crumbs
11. Single-Sip Cup Drinking
12. Kisses
13. Sponge-Balsa-Tongue Depressor
14. Tongue Depressor for Lip Closure - Production Criteria for / m, b, p /

13

# TARGET PHONEMES - / f, v /

**Oral Placement Components**

| | |
|---|---|
| **Jaw Height:** | **High** |
| **Tongue Position:** | **Retracted** |
| **Lips:** | **Lower Lip Retraction** |

**Suggested Activities:**

**Note:** The following techniques will improve placement and movement skills for the production of / f, v /. Not every client will need to use all of the activities. Some activities may be eliminated because the client already demonstrates the "Criteria for Success." A typical therapy session of 30 to 45 minutes will include five activities in addition to traditional speech therapy techniques.

1. Establishing a Natural Bite
2. Bite Block (Jaw Height Level #2)
3. Twin Bite Blocks for Symmetrical Jaw Stability (Jaw Height Level #2)
4. Bite Block for Jaw Stability (Jaw Height Level #2)
5. Gum Chewing
6. Bubble Blowing
7. Horn Blowing
8. Straw Drinking
9. Sponge-Balsa-Tongue Depressor
10. Tongue Depressor for Lip Closure
11. Cheerio for Lower Lip Retraction - Production Criteria for / f, v /

# TARGET PHONEMES - / θ (th), ð (th) /

**Oral Placement Components**

| | |
|---|---|
| **Jaw Height:** | Medium |
| **Tongue Position:** | Protruded |
| **Lips:** | Open |

**Suggested Activities:**

**Note:** The following techniques will improve placement and movement skills for the production of / θ (th), ð (th) /.

Not every client will need to use all of the activities. Some activities may be eliminated because the client already demonstrates the "Criteria for Success." A typical therapy session of 30 to 45 minutes will include five activities in addition to traditional speech therapy techniques.

1. Establishing a Natural Bite
2. Bite Block (Jaw Height Levels #2 - #7)
3. Twin Bite Blocks for Symmetrical Jaw Stability (Jaw Height Levels #2 - #7)
4. Bite Block for Jaw Stability (Jaw Height Levels #2 - #7)
5. Gum Chewing
6. Tongue Blade Protrusion - Production Criteria for / θ (th), ð (th) /

# TARGET PHONEMES - / t, d, n, l /

**Oral Placement Components**

| | |
|---|---|
| **Jaw Height:** | **Medium** |
| **Tongue Position:** | **Tongue-Tip Elevation** |
| **Lips:** | **Open** |

**Suggested Activities:**

**Note:** The following techniques will improve placement and movement skills for the production of / t, d, n, l /. Not every client will need to use all of the activities. Some activities may be eliminated because the client already demonstrates the "Criteria for Success." A typical therapy session of 30 to 45 minutes will include five activities in addition to traditional speech therapy techniques.

1. Establishing a Natural Bite
2. Bite Block (Jaw Height Levels #2 - #7)
3. Twin Bite Blocks for Symmetrical Jaw Stability (Jaw Height Levels #2 - #7)
4. Bite Block for Jaw Stability (Jaw Height Levels #2 - #7)
5. Gum Chewing
6. Bubble Blowing
7. Horn Blowing
8. Straw Drinking
9. Golf Ball Air Hockey
10. Blade Retraction with Resistance
11. Tongue-Tip Lateralization
12. Tongue-Tip Pointing
13. Cheerio for Tongue-Tip Elevation - Production Criteria for / t, d, n, l /

# TARGET PHONEMES - / k, g /

**Oral Placement Components**

| | |
|---|---|
| **Jaw Height:** | Low |
| **Tongue Position:** | Tongue-Tip Depression |
| **Lips:** | Open |

**Suggested Activities:**

**Note:** The following techniques will improve placement and movement skills for the production of / k, g /. Not every client will need to use all of the activities. Some activities may be eliminated because the client already demonstrates the "Criteria for Success." A typical therapy session of 30 to 45 minutes will include five activities in addition to traditional speech therapy techniques.

1. Establishing a Natural Bite
2. Bite Block (Jaw Height Levels #2 - #7)
3. Twin Bite Blocks for Symmetrical Jaw Stability (Jaw Height Levels #2 - #7)
4. Bite Block for Jaw Stability (Jaw Height Levels #2 - #7)
5. Gum Chewing
6. Bubble Blowing
7. Horn Blowing
8. Straw Drinking
9. Golf Ball Air Hockey
10. Blade Retraction with Resistance
11. Tongue-Tip Lateralization
12. Tongue-Tip Pointing
13. Cheerio for Tongue-Tip Depression - Production Criteria for / k, g /

# TARGET PHONEMES - / s, z /

**Oral Placement Components**

    **Jaw Height:**          High

    **Tongue Position:**          **Tongue-Tip Elevation/Depression**

    **Lips:**          Open

**Suggested Activities:**

**Note:** The following techniques will improve placement and movement skills for the production of / s, z /. Not every client will need to use all of the activities. Some activities may be eliminated because the client already demonstrates the "Criteria for Success." A typical therapy session of 30 to 45 minutes will include five activities in addition to traditional speech therapy techniques.

1. Establishing a Natural Bite
2. Bite Block (Jaw Height Levels #2 - #7)
3. Twin Bite Blocks for Symmetrical Jaw Stability (Jaw Height Levels #2 - #7)
4. Bite Block for Jaw Stability (Jaw Height Levels #2 - #7)
5. Gum Chewing
6. Bubble Blowing
7. Horn Blowing
8. Straw Drinking
9. Golf Ball Air Hockey
10. Blade Retraction with Resistance
11. Tongue-Tip Lateralization
12. Tongue-Tip Pointing
13. Cheerio for Tongue-Tip Elevation
14. Cheerio for Tongue-Tip Depression
15. Tongue-Tip Up and Down - Production Criteria for / s, z /

# TARGET PHONEMES - / ʃ(sh), ʧ(ch), ʤ(j) /

**Oral Placement Components**

| | |
|---|---|
| **Jaw Height:** | **High** |
| **Tongue Position:** | **Tongue-Tip Elevation  and Back of Tongue Side Spread** |
| **Lips:** | **Rounded/Protruded** |

**Suggested Activities:**

**Note:**  The following techniques will improve placement and movement skills for the production of / ʃ(sh), ʧ(ch), ʤ(j) /.  Not every client will need to use all of the activities.  Some activities may be eliminated because the client already demonstrates the "Criteria for Success."  A typical therapy session of 30 to 45 minutes will include five activities in addition to traditional speech therapy techniques.

1. Establishing a Natural Bite
2. Bite Block (Jaw Height Levels #2 - #7)
3. Twin Bite Blocks for Symmetrical Jaw Stability (Jaw Height Levels #2 - #7)
4. Bite Block for Jaw Stability (Jaw Height Levels #2 - #7)
5. Gum Chewing
6. Bubble Blowing
7. Horn Blowing
8. Straw Drinking
9. Golf Ball Air Hockey
10. Blade Retraction with Resistance
11. Tongue-Tip Lateralization
12. Tongue-Tip Pointing
13. Cheerio for Tongue-Tip Elevation
14. Cheerio for Tongue-Tip Depression
15. Tongue-Tip Up and Down
16. "EE" - Tongue Position Production Criteria for / ʃ(sh), ʧ(ch), ʤ(j) /.

# TARGET PHONEMES - / r, vocalic r /

**Oral Placement Components**

| | |
|---|---|
| **Jaw Height:** | **Medium or High** |
| **Tongue Position:** | **Back of Tongue Side Spread** |
| **Lips:** | **Lower Lip Protrusion/Tension** |

**Suggested Activities:**

**Note:** The following techniques will improve placement and movement skills for the production of / r, vocalic r /. Not every client will need to use all of the activities. Some activities may be eliminated because the client already demonstrates the "Criteria for Success." A typical therapy session of 30 to 45 minutes will include five activities in addition to traditional speech therapy techniques.

1. Establishing a Natural Bite
2. Bite Block (Jaw Height Levels #2 - #7)
3. Twin Bite Blocks for Symmetrical Jaw Stability (Jaw Height Levels #2 - #7)
4. Bite Block for Jaw Stability (Jaw Height Levels #2 - #7)
5. Gum Chewing
6. Bubble Blowing
7. Horn Blowing
8. Straw Drinking
9. Golf Ball Air Hockey
10. Tongue Depressor for Lip Closure
11. Blade Retraction with Resistance
12. Tongue-Tip Lateralization
13. Tongue-Tip Pointing
14. Cheerio for Tongue-Tip Elevation
15. Cheerio for Tongue-Tip Depression
16. Tongue-Tip Up and Down
17. "EE"
18. Dinosaur for / r / - Production Criteria for / r / and the vocalic / r /

# VOWEL SOUND PRODUCTION

Prior to initiating any articulation therapy program, it is critical that you determine the causative factors of the error sound production. If there is a placement and/or movement deficit, the technique described in the beginning of Chapter 3 should help you to make that determination. However, before you can initiate an OPT program directed towards improving vowel production, you must understand the relationship among the oral articulators during standard vowel production.

Let's begin by identifying the primary articulator in vowel sound production: the jaw, the lips or the tongue. Your first inclination may be to say, "the tongue." Before you make any decision, however, try something. Stand facing a mirror. Put your tongue tip down at midline behind your lower front teeth. Freeze your tongue in that position. Try not to move it. Now look in the mirror as you say the following vowels in isolation, slowly with a one-second pause between each vowel production: / ɪ (ih), ɛ (eh), ɑ (ah)./ What moved the most? The jaw, the lips or the tongue? The answer: the jaw. Now open your mouth to say "ah" and keep it open. Without moving your jaw but allowing your tongue to move freely, say the same vowels: This is not to say that the lips and tongue are not involved in vowel production, but I hope this demonstration showed you that the jaw is also a primary characteristic of vowel sound production.

Many of our clients evidence vowel distortions secondary to lack of jaw stability and jaw grading. Lip and tongue placement are secondary to jaw placement. During the administration of the articulation test, watch your client. If the jaw is not moving in a controlled, graded manner, there may be a placement and/or movement component to the pattern of vowel distortions. In some cases, there is a placement and movement disorder and a phonetic, phonological, or motor-planning disorder. To address one area of deficit, while ignoring the other, will negatively impact on your therapeutic success. You must address both the placement and/or movement deficit and the speech component (phonetic, phonological, or motor planning).

# PLACEMENT AND MOVEMENT Components of Vowel Sounds

| Phoneme | Jaw Height | Tongue Position | Lips | Voicing | Resonance |
|---------|-----------|-----------------|------|---------|-----------|
| ε (egg) | Medium | Retracted | Open | Yes | Oral |
| ʌ (up) | Medium | Retracted | Open | Yes | Oral |
| ʊ (good) | High | Retracted<br>Back of Tongue: Side Spread | Rounded | Yes | Oral |
| εi (aim) | Medium, Transition to High | Retracted<br>Back of Tongue: Side Spread | Open | Yes | Oral |
| ə (the) | Medium | Retracted | Open | Yes | Oral |
| O (own) | Medium, Transition to High | Retracted | Rounded | Yes | Oral |
| ɪ (his) | High | Retracted<br>Back of Tongue: Side Spread | Retracted | Yes | Oral |
| a (father) | Low | Retracted | Open | Yes | Oral |
| ɔ (off) | Medium | Retracted | Rounded | Yes | Oral |
| i (eat) | High | Retracted<br>Back of Tongue: Side Spread | Retracted | Yes | Oral |
| u (to) | High | Retracted<br>Back of Tongue: Side Spread | Rounded | Yes | Oral |
| æ (ask) | Low | Retracted | Open | Yes | Oral |

# TARGET PHONEMES - / I ( ih ), i ( ee ), u ( oo - as in shoe ), ʊ ( oo - as in good ) /

**Oral Placement Components**

| | |
|---|---|
| **Jaw Height:** | **High** |
| **Tongue Position:** | **Back of Tongue Side Spread** |
| **Lips:** | I, i  =  **Open** |
| | u,  ʊ  =  **Rounded** |

**Suggested Activities:**

**Note:** The following techniques will improve placement and movement skills for the production of / I, i, u, ʊ /. Not every client will need to use all of the activities. Some activities may be eliminated because the client already demonstrates the "Criteria for Success." A typical therapy session of 30 to 45 minutes will include five activities in addition to traditional speech therapy techniques.

1. Establishing a Natural Bite
2. Bite Block (Jaw Height Level #2)
3. Twin Bite Blocks for Symmetrical Jaw Stability (Jaw Height Level #2)
4. Bite Block for Jaw Stability (Jaw Height Level #2)
5. Gum Chewing
6. Bubble Blowing
7. Horn Blowing
8. Straw Drinking
9. "OO-EE"
10. "EE"

# TARGET PHONEMES - / ʌ ( uh - as in "up" ), O, ə (uh as in "the"), ɔ (aw), ɛ (eh) /

**Oral Placement Components**

| | |
|---|---|
| **Jaw Height:** | **Medium** |
| **Tongue Position:** | **Retracted** |
| **Lips:** | ʌ , ə , ɛ **= Open** |
| | O , ɔ **= Rounded** |

**Suggested Activities:**

**Note:** The following techniques will improve placement and movement skills for the production of / ʌ, ə, ɛ, O, ɔ /. Not every client will need to use all of the activities. Some activities may be eliminated because the client already demonstrates the "Criteria for Success." A typical therapy session of 30 to 45 minutes will include five activities in addition to traditional speech therapy techniques.

1.  Establishing a Natural Bite
2.  Bite Block (Jaw Height Levels #2 - #5)
3.  Twin Bite Blocks for Symmetrical Jaw Stability (Jaw Height Levels #2 - #5)
4.  Bite Block for Jaw Stability (Jaw Height Levels #2 - #5)
5.  Gum Chewing
6.  Bubble Blowing
7.  Horn Blowing
8.  Straw Drinking
9.  "OO-EE-AH"

# TARGET PHONEMES - / æ ( a - as in "ask"), a  ( a - as in "father" ) /

**Oral Placement Components**

| | |
|---|---|
| **Jaw Height:** | **Low** |
| **Tongue Position:** | **Retracted** |
| **Lips:** | **Open** |

**Suggested Activities:**

**Note:** The following techniques will improve placement and movement skills for the production of / æ, a /.  Not every client will need to use all of the activities.  Some activities may be eliminated because the client already demonstrates the "Criteria for Success."  A typical therapy session of 30 to 45 minutes will include five activities in addition to traditional speech therapy techniques.

1.  Bite Block (Jaw Height Levels #5 - #7)

2.  Twin Bite Blocks for Symmetrical Jaw Stability (Jaw Height Levels #5 - #7)

3.  Bite Block for Jaw Stability (Jaw Height Levels #5 - #7)

4. Gum Chewing

# CHAPTER 4
# PHONATION ACTIVITIES

Before you begin to use any of the activities in this chapter, please make sure you have read the information in Chapters 1 and 2. The information given there is so important it may be the difference between success and failure for you and for your client. Remember, that maintaining a stable posture throughout the completion of each **Phonation Activity** will be required for maximum success during your therapy session, as well as during the implementation of homework assignments.

In my classes, I show a video of a five-year-old boy with cerebral palsy who has been referred to me for a assessment. There is a difference of opinion as to what the goals should be for this young man as he enters the public school system. He has been receiving private speech therapy for four years.

One speech-language pathologist suggests the following:
1. Increase receptive and expressive language
2. Increase sentence length
3. Improve the production of / s /

The other speech-language pathologist suggests:

1. Improve abdominal grading
2. Speak on exhalation only
3. Improve jaw stability
4. Improve lip closure
5. Improve tongue retraction

We then observe the video of this very intelligent five-year-old having a conversation with me about Christmas. His language skills appear to be age appropriate. Without testing we cannot be sure, but he is certainly able to talk about complex ideas and issues. What is also obvious is that he is:

1. Speaking on a combination of inhalation and exhalation
2. Using a compensatory body posture to push out the air
3. Running out of air before he can finish a thought
4. Choosing to speak in two to three-syllable utterances rather than using longer phrases. We hear him say only one six-syllable utterance, which he is only able to do by placing his entire body in exaggerated extension to push out the air.
5. Demonstrating jaw sliding, insufficient lip closure, and excessive tongue protrusion during conversational speech
6. Drooling

So, what should our goals be? From a motor speech perspective , we are obligated to choose the second set of goals, the ones suggested by the school-based speech-language pathologist. Did you think those were from the private therapist? There is a misconception in our field that the best therapists are in private practice. Over the past thirty-six years I have worked with SLPs in schools, clinics, hospitals, early intervention programs, and in private practice. In my personal experience, quality is not based on the "setting" in which we work. If I were to write the goals for the same child, I would write them to reflect the goals of each of

26

these therapists because their goals for this child are the same; only their methods vary. Here is my set of goals for my five-year-old client:

1. Improve abdominal grading to enable Stevie to increase sentence length
2. Speak on exhalation only by learning to inhale before each breath group
3. Improve jaw stability for improved feeding skills and for phoneme production
4. Improve lip closure for improved production of bilabial speech sounds
5. Improve tongue retraction for improved production of the phoneme /s/

With this particular child, and others like him, we should begin with the activities of **"Phonation."** Refer to the Sample Program Plan on page 204 to find the activities for feeding and speech which were written into his IEP.

We will also use these activities with clients who have any or all of the following goals:

1. Improve awareness of the lips as a prerequisite for lip closure for feeding, speech clarity and drooling control
2. Improve abdominal grading to support controlled oral airflow for functional oral language
3. Teach the association of airflow and oral movements as a component of phoneme imitation
4. Teach supported directionality of oral airflow for improved velopharyngeal functioning
5. Improve jaw grading for jaw-lip-tongue dissociation
6. Improve lip closure, protrusion, retraction and lower lip retraction/protrusion for standard speech sound production
7. Improve tongue grading for retraction, tip-elevation/depression, back of tongue side spread, and standard speech sound production

**Note:**   Each activity in this chapter will identify which of the previous goals you will be addressing.

27

# BUBBLE BLOWING HIERARCHY

This activity is designed to teach clients to use controlled, elongated oral airflow as a component of speech clarity. Therapeutic bubble blowing requires abdominal grading, jaw stability, lip rounding and tongue retraction. Each of these skills is needed for speech sound production. For non-verbal clients, Bubble Blowing teaches how oral air can be used to make something happen. Once this concept is understood, teaching imitation of speech sounds becomes a lot easier. Bubble Blowing is also helpful for working with those clients who are speaking on inhalation or are using a combination of inhalation and exhalation.

The specific oral placement or movement goals are listed after each Step.

Suggestions:

1. Try to limit bubbles to oral placement techniques. If they are used for reinforcement for other tasks, the motivation to work may be eliminated, or the client may want to swat at the bubbles, thereby, removing the hands from midline.

2. As in all OPT work, the client must be placed in a stable posture. For some clients, Bubble Blowing will be impossible if attempted in a seated posture. Clients who do not have postural stability in a chair and who are "fixing" to stabilize should begin this activity in a **supine** position on an incline mat (wedge).

3. You will need a Bubble Tube, a Bubble Bear and a puppet to implement this activity. Use good quality bubbles that do not pop too easily. You want the bubbles to last until the client can coordinate the oral movements with appropriate airflow.

4. Monitor to ensure that the client is not using compensatory body postures (e.g., shoulder elevation, whole body extension, high or low jaw fixing).

5. The therapist must hold the wand or the Bubble Bear throughout this activity.

6. Hold the wand approximately one inch from the client's mouth.

7. Each step must be completed 10 times (10 repetitions) before going onto the next step.

8. Each step of this activity should be done in rapid repetitions without a break.

9. Visually Impaired Clients: Bubbles can be used if there is only minimal response to light. Work in a dark room with a flashlight shining on the bubble. The movement of the bubble will be highlighted.

10. Homework: During each session, establish where the client fails on the hierarchy (e.g., at Step #3 the client can blow 5 times successfully). Practice that step at the highest level of successful repetitions.

Step #1
1. The therapist blows a bubble ("existing bubble") and catches it on the wand.
2. Pop the existing bubble on the client's open mouth, as pictured below:

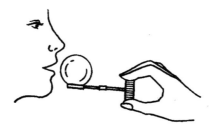

3. Wait for any oral movement response (i.e., oral movement or anticipation of movement).
4. Continue this technique if the client's tongue protrudes and then retracts to effect lip closure. Discontinue this technique if the client's tongue protrudes but does not retract, despite assisted jaw elevation.
5. Continue if any lip movement or jaw elevation is achieved.
6. <u>Criteria for Success:</u>  Repeat 10 times or until you are sure the client feels the sensation consistently on the surface of the lips.

<u>Goals:</u>
   1. Develop awareness of sensation on the lips as a prerequisite for lip closure for feeding, speech and drooling control
   2. Achieve lip closure from an open mouth posture.

<u>Target Phonemes:</u> / m, b, p /

Step #2
1. The therapist blows a bubble and catches it on a wand.
2. Hold the wand 1" horizontally in front of the client's mouth.
3. Place your other hand on the client's abdomen for increased awareness of abdominal involvement during exhalation (i.e., adding weight).
4. As the client exhales, press gently on the abdominal muscles in response to the exhalation.
5. Reward the client for any movement of the bubble on the wand.
6. <u>Criteria for Success:</u>  Repeat 10 times, without a break, before going on to Step #3.

<u>Goals:</u>
   1. Associate abdominal exhalation with movement of the bubble
   2. Develop controlled oral airflow for phoneme production

<u>Target Phoneme:</u> / h /

### Step #3

1. The therapist blows a bubble and catches it on the wand.
2. Hold the wand horizontally 1" in front of the client's mouth.
3. With your other hand, assist with jaw stability and lip rounding. Place your palm under the client's jaw. Use your 5 fingers to pull forward gently on the cheeks, as picture below. This support posture will allow the client to volitionally constrict the orbicularis-oris muscles for controlled airflow.

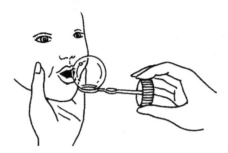

4. Instruct the client to blow the bubble off the wand.
5. <u>Criteria for Success:</u> Repeat 10 times, without a break, before going on to Step #4.
   <u>Goals:</u>
      1. Improve controlled oral airflow volume
      2. Work on jaw-lip dissociation
      3. Develop strength and stability in the orbicularis-oris muscles for lip rounding

   <u>Target Phonemes:</u> / w, o, u, ʊ, ɔ, ʃ (sh), tʃ (ch), dʒ (j) /

### Step #4

1. Dip the wand into the bubble solution.
2. Hold the wand vertically 1" in front of the client's mouth.
3. Continue to use assisted jaw and/or lip stability if necessary.
   **Note:** For some clients a 2" cut piece of a jumbo diameter straw can be used to transition from assisted lip rounding to independent lip rounding.
4. <u>Criteria for Success:</u> Blow bubbles 10 times in this position, without a break, before going onto Step #5.
   <u>Goals:</u>
      1. Improve controlled, elongated oral airflow
      2. Work on jaw-lip dissociation
      3. Improve lip rounding skills

   <u>Target Phonemes:</u> / w, o, u, ʊ, ɔ, ʃ (sh), tʃ (ch), dʒ (j) /

Step #5

1. Use a Bubble Bear or other oval-shaped wand.
2. Teach the client to use a whispered "hoo" position to blow. You should be able to hear a voiceless "hoo." Working in this posture will ensure jaw stability and dissociated lip rounding; it will also keep the cheeks (masseter muscles) tight.
3. Hold the wand vertically 1" in front of the client's mouth.
4. Instruct the client to blow through the Bubble Bear wand, using the whispered "hoo" position, as pictured below.

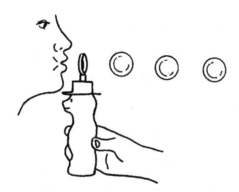

5. Criteria for Success: Blow bubbles 10 times in this position before going onto Step #6.

Goals:
1. Improve controlled, elongated oral airflow
2. Develop jaw stability
3. Achieve jaw-lip dissociation
4. Improve lip rounding/protrusion skills

Target Phonemes: / w, o, u, ʊ, ɔ, ʃ (sh), tʃ (ch), dʒ (j) /

Step #6

1. Use a Bubble Bear or other oval-shaped wand.
2. Hold the wand 1" in front of the client's mouth.
3. Work in the whispered "hoo" position; eliminate all therapist-assisted jaw and/or lip stability.
4. Talk about using rounded lips and how these rounded lips "feel" as the client blows the bubbles.
5. Criteria for Success: Blow bubbles 10 times in rapid succession, without a break, with appropriate jaw stability and lip rounding (jaw-lip dissociation) before going on to Step #7.

Goals:

1. Improve controlled, elongated oral airflow
2. Establish jaw-lip dissociation
3. Develop lip protrusion skills
4. Improve tongue retraction skills
5. To work on jaw-lip-tongue dissociation

Target Phonemes: / w, o, u, ʊ, ɔ, ʃ (sh), ʧ (ch), ʤ (j) /

## Step #7

1. Use a Bubble Bear or other oval-shaped wand.
2. Introduce a puppet with a mouth that opens and closes (who likes to eat bubbles).
3. Hold the wand 1" in front of the client's mouth.
4. Hold the puppet 18" in front of the client.
5. Instruct the client to blow in the whispered "hoo" position.
6. The puppet will eat the bubbles only if they reach its mouth.
7. Criteria for Success: Repeat this task 10 times before going onto Step #8.

   Goals:

   1. Improve controlled, elongated oral airflow (abdominal grading)
   2. Achieve jaw-lip dissociation
   3. Improve lip protrusion skills
   4. Maintain tongue retraction skills
   5. Develop jaw-lip-tongue dissociation

   Target Phonemes: / w, o, u, ʊ, ɔ, ʃ (sh), ʧ (ch), ʤ (j) /

## Step #8

1. Repeat Step #7, increasing the distance of the puppet from the client's mouth to 2 feet. Maintain the criteria of 10 successful repetitions before progressing to #2 (below).
2. Increase the distance by 6" inches as each set of 10 successful repetitions is achieved.
3. Criteria for Success: Using 6" inch increments, work up to the child blowing bubbles 4 feet from the Bubble Bear's wand.

   **Note:** The wand remains held stable 1" in front of the client's mouth. The client will blow the bubbles the length of 4 feet.

Goals:

1. Improve controlled, elongated oral airflow (abdominal grading)
2. Improve jaw-lip dissociation
3. Improve lip protrusion skills
4. Maintain tongue retraction skills
5. Achieve jaw-lip-tongue dissociation

Target Phonemes: / w, o, u, ʊ, ɔ, ʃ (sh), ʧ (ch), ʤ (j) /

**Note:** *Bubbles as Therapy Tools*, by Sara Rosenfeld-Johnson, SLP, is a one-hour video designed to teach this OPT technique to therapists, parents, teachers, etc.

# "AH" IN SUPINE ( or "Up-Up-Up Tickle")

This activity can be used for a variety of client needs.  I have found it to be very helpful in working with children who have:

1. Insufficient oral airflow, volume and duration.
2. The diagnosis of Autism, PDD or Asperger's Syndrome who are not imitating phonemes but benefit from firm touch to control behavior and to target volitional movements.
3. An inability to imitate isolated phonemes consistently.
4. Difficulty understanding turn taking.

The client should be positioned using a wedge.  The position of the client on the wedge will stabilize the lower portion of the body, the back and the head to allow the therapist to work directly on the abdominal muscles. Many of our clients do not understand that exhalation of air, paired with vocalizations, are the necessary components of  phoneme or word imitation.  This technique will address these components.

The specific oral placement or movement goals are listed after each Step.


Suggestions:

1. You will need a 45-degree angled wedge which is approximately two feet high at the back to implement this activity.  Always work on the floor or on a mat.
2. If your goal is to associate abdominal exhalation with blowing, use the position pictured on the next page to teach Bubble Blowing or Horn Blowing.  I also strongly recommend consultation with an occupational therapist or a physical therapist who can help you with movements to stimulate controlled exhalations, is also strongly recommended. Therapists trained in gross motor positioning or Neuro-Developmental Technique (NDT) can be helpful in this area if you feel you need additional guidance.
3. Two other simple positions to facilitate exhalation with clients who do not have adequate abdominal support are:
   a. Prone on a therapy ball.
   b. Sitting the client on a therapy ball or large chair, couch, or end of a bed. The therapist or parent is positioned behind the client to provide rotation.
4. If you are unsure how to position the client, I recommend consultation with an occupational therapist or a physical therapist.
5. Do this activity only if the client enjoys being tickled.
6. This technique can be used to teach "eye-to-mouth contact." As OPT therapists, we

want the client looking at our mouth to gain further information, rather than at our eyes.

7. Since the position described in this technique limits extraneous stimuli, and is therefore a favorite of children with Sensory Processing Difficulties (including clients with the diagnosis of Autism, PDD and Asperger's Syndrome), I will occasionally continue to work in this position after my initial goals have been met, at the client's request. Work in a quiet room with low light when implementing this technique with these clients to reduce external stimuli which may be distracting.

8. <u>Homework:</u> Because of the complexity of this technique, homework assignments should be made on a case-by-case basis.

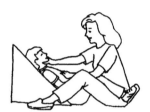

<u>Step #1</u>

1. Establish where the client is ticklish (the "tickle-spot"). An audible laugh must accompany the response.
2. Place the client on his/her back on the wedge. The client's bottom will be on the floor or mat where you are working. For the moment, the client's legs will be flat or bent.
3. Position your body on the floor or mat facing the client. Use your bent legs to support the sides of the client's body. The client's legs will then either be bent over your body or will remain flat, depending on their size. Your arms should remain free to complete the technique.
4. Begin with both of your hands on the client's abdominal muscles.
5. As you work up the body to the tickle spot, say "Up, up, up." Continue to the tickle spot as long as the client maintains "eye-to-mouth contact." If the client looks away, return to the original starting location on the abdominal muscles and wait for renewed "eye-to-mouth contact."
6. When you reach the tickle spot, tickle the client. Immediately place one of your palms on the client's abdominal muscles to add awareness of where the air is coming from. Use the thumb on your other hand to pull down gently on the client's jaw. This change in jaw position should result in the production of the phoneme "ah." Work on imitation of this phoneme. Transition to other phonemes by using your fingers to change the position of the client's articulators (Facial Cueing).

7. An "Echo Horn" can also be used to associate turn taking with imitation. Transition from the hand placement on the abdominal muscles to holding the Echo Horn in front of the client's mouth as he/she vocalizes. Move the Echo Horn to your mouth as you imitate what the child is saying or to change the vocal stimuli.

Goals:

1. Minimize superficial external stimuli in an attempt to gain client attention (availability for learning)
2. Associate abdominal grading with oral airflow
3. Associate abdominal grading with oral airflow and vocalizations as a component of learing to imitate phonemes.

# CANDLE BLOWING

This activity is designed to teach controlled, elongated oral airflow. Cake "A" will be used to increase volitional oral airflow and duration. Cake "B" will address clients who have inhalation/exhalation confusion or clients who need to learn to speak in shorter breath groups to eliminate the compensatory habit of speaking on residual air.

Blowing out the candles on a child's birthday cake can be a wonderful experience or a very painful one. Many of our clients who do not have the necessary oral airflow (abdominal grading) or the motor-planning skills to perform this "easy" task are devastated at their own parties. I have worked with parents who are equally devastated at their child's difficulties. Teaching this task prior to the actual birthday celebration addresses these social, emotional needs. It also works directly on improving volitional oral airflow and duration for functional connected speech development.

The specific oral placement or movement goals are listed after each "Step."

Suggestions:

1. Since candle blowing can be dangerous if the client touches the fire, work with an assistant until the rules of candle blowing are mastered.
2. You will need a "cake," a box of matches, one large candle and a box of small tapered candles to implement this activity.
3. Place a lit candle on your desk to be used to re-light your stimuli candles.
4. Make the "cake" prior to the introduction of this technique.
   a. Use a piece of Styrofoam or cardboard box the size of a sheet cake, 2" to 3 inches deep.
   b. Cover the Styrofoam or box with tin foil to prevent a fire.
   c. Decorate the cake with the same items that will be on the "real" cake. This will prevent too much excitement on the part of the client which could result in reduced skill levels on the day of the party.

5. Each step must be completed 10 times (10 repetitions), without a break, before going onto the next Step.
6. All repetitions should be done rapidly.
7. Monitor to ensure that the client is not using compensatory body postures (e.g., shoulder elevation, whole body leaning, high or low jaw fixing).
8. Prerequisite: Bubble Blowing Hierarchy." Complete the Criteria for Success in Step #4.

37

9. Homework: During the session, establish where the client fails on the hierarchy (e.g., at Step #1 the client can blow 5 times successfully). Practice that Step at the highest level of successful repetitions.

## CAKE "A"

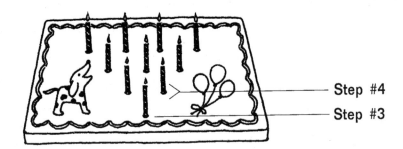

Step#1

1. Work at seated upright mouth level. The client's mouth should be at the level of the candle. The client should not have to blow down to extinguish the candle.
2. Light a large candle and hold it 4 inches in front of the client's mouth.
3. Instruct the client to blow out the candle without moving his/her body closer to the flame. If the client does not know how to blow volitionally, stop this activity and return to "Bubble Blowing" or to "Ah" in Supine.
4. Use assisted jaw stability and/or assisted lip rounding if necessary: Place the palm of your non-dominant hand under the client's jaw. Use your 5 fingers to pull forward gently on the cheeks. This support will allow the client to volitionally constrict the orbicularis-oris muscles for controlled oral airflow.
5. <u>Criteria for Success:</u> Repeat 10 times before going on to Step #2.
   <u>Goals:</u>
   1. Associate abdominal exhalation with volitional airflow
   2. Improved abdominal grading
   3. Achieve jaw-lip dissociation
   4. Improve agility and placement of the orbicularis-oris muscles for lip rounding

<u>Target Phonemes:</u> / w, o, u, ʊ, ɔ, ʃ (sh), tʃ (ch), dʒ (j) /

Step #2

1. Work at seated upright mouth level.
2. Transition to a small, tapered candle (e.g., Hanukkah Candle) which burns slowly so it can be re-lit many times and does not drip.

3. Present the candle 4 inches in front of the client's mouth.

4. Instruct the client to blow out the candle.

5. Use assisted jaw and lip stability if necessary.

6. Criteria for Success:  Repeat 10 times before going on to Step #3.

   Goals:

   1. Associate abdominal exhalation with volitional airflow

   2. Improve abdominal grading

   3. Achieve jaw-lip dissociation

   4. Improve placement for lip rounding

Target Phonemes:  / w, o, u, ʊ, ɔ,  ʃ (sh),  ʧ (ch),  ʤ (j) /

## Step #3

1. Work at seated upright mouth level.

2. Place one small candle in the cake as pictured previously (Cake "A").

3. Hold the cake with the single candle 4 inches in front of the client's mouth.

4. Instruct the client to blow out the candle.

5. Use assisted jaw and lip stability if necessary.

6. Criteria for Success:  Repeat 10 times before going on to Step #4.

   Goals:

   1. Associate abdominal exhalation with volitional airflow

   2. Improve abdominal grading

   3. Achieve jaw-lip dissociation

   4. Improve placement for lip rounding

Target Phonemes:  / w, o, u, ʊ, ɔ,  ʃ (sh),  ʧ (ch),  ʤ (j) /

## Step #4

1. Work at seated upright mouth level.

2. Add two small candles to the cake (three candles in all) as pictured previously.

3. Instruct the client to breathe in and then to blow out all three candles.  You may have to work on inhalation/exhalation control at this time.  Place your flat palm on the client's abdomen.  Rest your hand on the abdominal muscles as the client inhales; push in gently as he/she exhales.

**Note:**

    a. For clients with motor planning difficulties, the use of a short straw or piece of tubing may be helpful. Once they are able to blow through the therapy tool, repeat this Step to transition from supported to independent blowing.

    b. If these suggestions are not sufficient enough to eliminate the confusion, refer to the Cake "B" techniques.

    c. If the client cannot sustain oral airflow with the required duration you may want to stop this activity, introduce the TalkTools® Duration Tube activity to teach duration. Once duration has been mastered you can return to Step #4 in this hierarchy.

4. Teach the whispered "hoo" position. Eliminate all assisted jaw and lip stability.

    **Note:** Refer to "Bubble Blowing" for a description of the whispered "hoo" position.

5. <u>Criteria for Success:</u> Repeat 10 times consecutively before going on to Step #5.

    <u>Goals:</u>

        1. Improve volitional airflow volume and duration
        2. Improve abdominal grading
        3. Improve jaw-lip dissociation
        4. Improve placement for lip rounding


<u>Target Phonemes:</u> / w, o, u, ʊ, ɔ, ʃ (sh), ʧ (ch), ʤ (j) /


<u>Step #5</u>

1. Work at seated upright mouth level.

2. Continue to add candles in rows as pictured previously, one row at a time.

3. Instruct the client to breathe in and then blow out all of the candles.

4. <u>Criteria for Success:</u> Repeat 10 times at each row level. Go on to Step #6 when the client can blow out all 10 candles with a single exhalation, 10 times consecutively.

    <u>Goals:</u>

        1. Improve volitional oral airflow volume and duration
        2. Improve abdominal grading
        3. Improve lip-jaw dissociation
        4. Improve placement for tongue retraction
        5. Achieve jaw-lip-tongue dissociation

    <u>Target Phonemes:</u> / w, o, u, ʊ, ɔ, ʃ (sh), ʧ (ch), ʤ (j) /

Step #6

1. Place the Styrofoam or cardboard cake on the table in front of the client as it would be placed at the real party.
2. Use the age equivalent number of candles in the appropriate configuration.
3. Instruct the client to breathe in and blow out all of the candles at once.
4. Criteria for Success: Repeat 10 times before the day of the birthday celebration.
    Goal: Transition to a more normal environment (placement of the cake on the table).

**Note:** If the client's birthday comes before you have completed the six Steps in this activity, disregard the age appropriate number of candles. Present the real cake with the number of candles that the child can blow out successfully in the appropriate configuration and height.

## Cake "B"

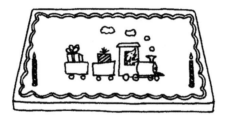

Step #1

1. Work at seated upright mouth level. The client's mouth should be at the level of the candle. The client should not have to blow down to extinguish the candle.
2. Light a large candle and present it 4 inches in front of the client's mouth.
3. Instruct the client to blow out the candle without moving his/her body closer to the flame. If the client does not know how to blow volitionally, stop this activity and return to "Bubble Blowing" or to "Ah" in Supine.
4. Use assisted jaw stability or lip rounding, if necessary. Place your palm under the client's jaw. Use your 5 fingers to pull forward gently on the cheeks. This support will allow the client to volitionally constrict the orbicularis-oris muscles for controlled airflow.
5. Criteria for Success: Repeat 10 times before going on to Step #2.
    Goals:
        1. Associate abdominal exhalation with volitional airflow
        2. Achieve jaw-lip dissociation
        3. Improve agility in the orbicularis-oris muscles for lip rounding placement.

Target Phonemes: / w, o, u, ʊ, ɔ, ʃ (sh), tʃ (ch), dʒ (j) /

Step #2

1. Work at seated upright mouth level.
2. Transition to a small, tapered candle (e.g., Hanukkah Candle) which burns slowly, so that it can be re-lit many times and does not drip.
3. Hold the candle 4 inches in front of the client's mouth.
4. Instruct the client to blow out the candle.
5. Use assisted jaw and lip stability if necessary.
6. Criteria for Success: Repeat 10 times consecutively before going on to Step #3.
    Goals:
       1. Associate abdominal exhalation with volitional airflow
       2. Achieve jaw-lip dissociation
       3. Improve placement for lip rounding
    Target Phonemes: / w, o, u, ʊ, ɔ, ʃ (sh), ʧ (ch), ʤ (j)/


Step #3

1. Work at seated upright mouth level.
2. Place one small candle in one end of the cake as pictured on the previous page (Cake "B").
3. Hold the cake with the single candle 4 inches in front of the client's mouth.
4. Instruct the client to blow out the candle.
5. Use assisted jaw and lip stability if necessary.
6. Criteria for Success: Repeat 10 times consecutively before going on to Step #4.
    Goals:
       1. Associate abdominal exhalation with volitional airflow
       2. Achieve jaw-lip dissociation
       3. Improve placement for lip rounding
    Target Phonemes: / w, o, u, ʊ, ɔ, ʃ (sh), ʧ (ch), ʤ (j) /


Step #4

1. Work at seated upright mouth level.
2. Add one small candle to the opposite end of the cake closest to the client's mouth.
3. Instruct the client to blow out the original candle and then to blow out the additional candle. The client will inhale automatically before attempting to blow out the second candle.
4. Repeat the same technique, but this time associate the words "inhale" or "breathe in" when the client is inhaling.

5.  Criteria for Success:  Repeat 10 times consecutively before going on to Step #5.
    Goals:

    1.  Associate abdominal exhalation with volitional airflow
    2.  Reduce the length of a breath group
    3.  Exhibit inhalation vs. exhalation
    4.  Improve jaw-lip dissociation
    5.  Improve placement for lip rounding

Target Phonemes:  / w, o, u, ʊ, ɔ,  ʃ (sh),  tʃ (ch),  ʤ (j) /

## Step #5

1.  Work at seated upright mouth level.
2.  Continue to use only the two candles placed at opposite ends of the cake.
3.  Instruct the client to blow out the original candle, inhale, and then produce a whispered "hoo" sound as he/she blows out the second candle.
4.  Criteria for Success:  Repeat 10 times consecutively before going on to Step #6.
    Goals:

    1.  Associate abdominal exhalation with volitional airflow
    2.  Associate exhalation with phonation

## Step #6

1.  Work at seated upright mouth level.
2.  Continue to use the same candle configuration.
3.  Instruct the client to blow out the original candle, inhale, and then produce a voiced "hoo" sound as he/she blows out the second candle.
4.  Criteria for Success:  Continue this technique, using a variety of plosive sound syllables (poo, too, koo, foo, soo) until the client understands that speech is produced only on exhaled air.
    Goals:

    1.  Associate abdominal exhalation with volitional airflow
    2.  Associate exhalation with phonation

## Step #7

1.  Repeat 4. in Step #6 using any three syllables.
2.  Transition this knowledge away from the cake, using a line chart as pictured below:

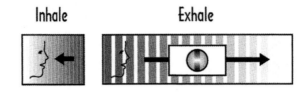

3. Instructions for how to use the line chart:
    a. Place any one-syllable item or picture card on the exhale segment of the line chart.
    b. Touch the inhale segment of the line chart as you say "inhale" and as the client inhales.
    c. Touch the exhale segment of the line chart as the client labels the item or picture card with the exhaled air.
4. <u>Criteria for Success:</u> Use 10 items or picture cards, in rapid succession without a break, as described previously.

    <u>Goal:</u> Learn that speech is produced only on exhaled air

# HORN BLOWING HIERARCHY
## Phonation and Articulation

The horns presented on this Airflow Hierarchy form represent a technique for improving abdominal muscle grading for prolongation of controlled exhalation. The #1 horn is the easiest to blow, while #12 is the hardest. The therapist should hold the horn perpendicular to the client's mouth and parallel to the floor. By allowing the client to hold the horn, you may facilitate any or all of the following compensatory problems:

1. Teeth biting on the mouthpiece for jaw stability, which will inhibit jaw-lip dissociation
2. Body extensor patterns which are associated with volitional hand-to-mouth movements in many of our clients
3. Bite reflex

Although each horn is presented as it relates to improving airflow and abdominal grading, horns are also a valuable tool for building awareness of the articulators, developing placement and control in specific muscles (abdominal, lips, tongue and jaw) and for reducing/ eliminating drooling. Using horns can be a part of the development of the following components of standard speech production:

1. Jaw grading
2. Jaw-lip dissociation
3. Jaw-tongue dissociation
4. Lip closure for saliva control (drooling)

5. Lip rounding
6. Tongue retraction
7. Back of tongue side spread
8. Motor planning/muscle memory

All horns from #9 through #12 are more difficult to blow. As lip protrusion is increased, tongue retraction will be initiated. These horns will address tongue retraction and grading, which are necessary components of all speech sound production with the exception of /θ - ð/. Use horns #9 through #12 for clients who do not have airflow deficits, but are working on the correction of an interdental or a lateral lisp.

45

# Oral Placement and Movement Goals

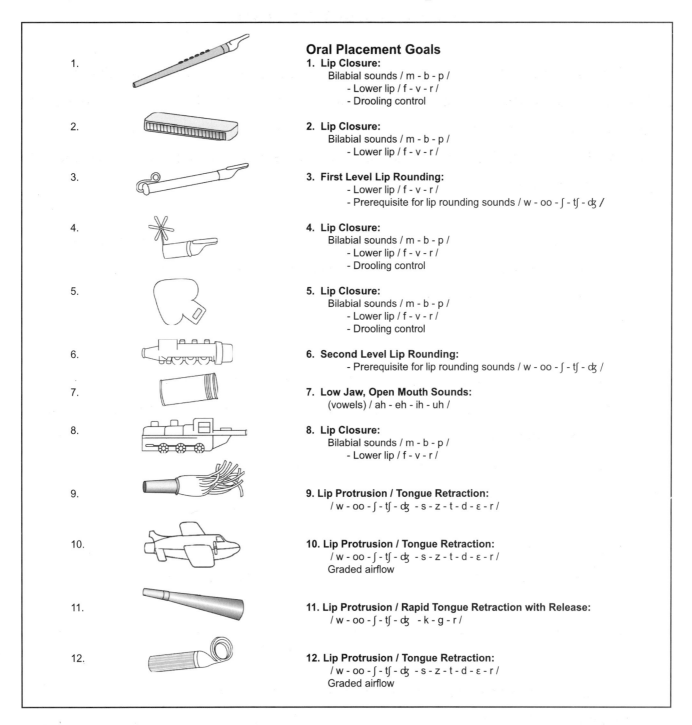

**Oral Placement Goals**

1. **Lip Closure:**
   Bilabial sounds / m - b - p /
   - Lower lip / f - v - r /
   - Drooling control

2. **Lip Closure:**
   Bilabial sounds / m - b - p /
   - Lower lip / f - v - r /

3. **First Level Lip Rounding:**
   - Lower lip / f - v - r /
   - Prerequisite for lip rounding sounds / w - oo - ʃ - tʃ - dʒ /

4. **Lip Closure:**
   Bilabial sounds / m - b - p /
   - Lower lip / f - v - r /
   - Drooling control

5. **Lip Closure:**
   Bilabial sounds / m - b - p /
   - Lower lip / f - v - r /
   - Drooling control

6. **Second Level Lip Rounding:**
   - Prerequisite for lip rounding sounds / w - oo - ʃ - tʃ - dʒ /

7. **Low Jaw, Open Mouth Sounds:**
   (vowels) / ah - eh - ih - uh /

8. **Lip Closure:**
   Bilabial sounds / m - b - p /
   - Lower lip / f - v - r /

9. **Lip Protrusion / Tongue Retraction:**
   / w - oo - ʃ - tʃ - dʒ - s - z - t - d - ɛ - r /

10. **Lip Protrusion / Tongue Retraction:**
    / w - oo - ʃ - tʃ - dʒ - s - z - t - d - ɛ - r /
    Graded airflow

11. **Lip Protrusion / Rapid Tongue Retraction with Release:**
    / w - oo - ʃ - tʃ - dʒ - k - g - r /

12. **Lip Protrusion / Tongue Retraction:**
    / w - oo - ʃ - tʃ - dʒ - s - z - t - d - ɛ - r /
    Graded airflow

**\*Note:** When a client relies on lip retraction to blow a horn, it may be a compensatory pattern to establish jaw stability. Go to a lower level on the hierarchy until the client can blow with abdominal constriction and lip closure, rounding or protrusion. Inhibit all compensatory body postures.

| #1 = any duration | #2 = 1 sec. | #3,4 = 1+ sec. |
| --- | --- | --- |
| #5, 6, 7, 8 = 2 sec. | #9, 10 = 2+ sec. | #11, 12 = 3 sec. |

Horn therapy has many benefits. It addresses deficits in abdominal grading, is a prerequisite for improving velopharyngeal functioning and targets specific speech sound placement. In combination with the Straw Drinking Hierarchy, it is a valuable technique for eliminating the primary physiological component of the interdental lisp: tongue protrusion and/or tongue thrusting.

The specific oral placement or movement goals are listed after each Step.

Suggestions:

1. Establish that the horns are therapy tools and should not be used as toys by either clients or their siblings. When not used for practice, these tools should be kept out of reach.

2. You will need the horns in the TalkTools® Original Horn Kit to implement this activity.

3. The therapist/parent must hold the horn to prevent the use of compensatory postures (biting or lip retraction). Once the technique is learned, it may be possible to allow the older client to hold the horn. It is critical to the success of this program that the client not bite on the horn as that posture will inhibit dissociation. The horns would then become toys.

4. Monitor to ensure the client is not using compensatory body postures (e.g., shoulder elevation, whole body extension, teeth biting or lip retraction).

5. Follow the horn hierarchy from Horn #1 through Horn #12 when your goal is to improve abdominal airflow for expanding utterance length. The horns in the kit are designed to increase abdominal muscle demand in very small increments to ensure success (Quest Engineering, 2007).

6. When you are working with a client who has motor-planning deficits, work through the entire hierarchy from Horn #1 through Horn #12 to facilitate labial (lip) placement, mobility and motor planning for lip movements.

7. Use the horns for specific speech sound teaching as described on the right side of the picture form. For example, if the targeted sound is "sh," begin at the lowest level horn for that sound. In this case, Horn #3 would be where you would begin.

   **Note:**

   a. Flat mouthed horns will target lip closure to address drooling control and for phonemes which require the following placement:

      1) lip approximation / m, b, p /

      2) lower lip retraction / f, v /

      3) lower lip protrusion / r and the vocalic r /

47

b. Round-mouthed horns will address placement for lip rounding phonemes.

c. The harder the client blows, the more tongue retraction you will facilitate.

8. Pay close attention to the duration requirements for each horn. The sound duration of the horn is critical to the success of this activity.

9. Each horn must be blown 25 times in rapid repetitions, using only lips and abdominal grading with no compensatory posturing, before proceeding to the next horn on the hierarchy. 25 repetitions ensures 1 repetition at the next horn level. This criteria should be met for any age client.

10. Jaw support and assisted lip closure may be used for Horn #1 and Horn #2. Beginning with Horn #3, no assisted jaw or lip support should be given.

11. You should never use two horns simultaneously. Once you have met the criteria for success (25 blows at the required duration), you will not go back to that horn.

12. Hearing Impaired Clients: Horns can be used successfully with this population, despite the fact that the client cannot "hear" the sound that the horn makes. Place a sound sensitive toy (e.g., a dancing plant) in front of the client. When the horn is blown, the sound sensitive toy will move to reinforce the task of successful blowing.

13. The video entitled *Horns as Therapy Tools* teaches this technique and the reasons for use as a part of an overall treatment plan. It is designed for therapists, parents, teachers, etc., to ensure that each step is introduced and practiced correctly.

14. Homework: Establish during the session where the client fails on the hierarchy (e.g., he/she can blow Horn #1, 8 times successfully with assisted jaw elevation and lip rounding). Practice that level daily for a minimum of one week.


Step #1

1. In this step you will determine which of the 12 horns in the TalkTools® Original Horn Kit you will use with each individual client.

2. Begin with Horn #1.

   **Note:** For this technique to be effective, the following sound duration criteria for each horn must be achieved before progressing to the next horn on the hierarchy.

| #1 = any duration | #2 = 1 sec. | #3,4 = 1+ sec. |
|---|---|---|
| #5, 6, 7, 8 = 2 sec. | #9, 10 = 2+ sec. | #11, 12 = 3 sec. |

3. Place the tip of the mouthpiece at midline on the client's lower lip as pictured below.

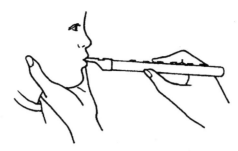

4. Instruct the client to blow the horn. One of the following scenarios will be observed:
    a. If the client is unable to blow the horn because of lack of sufficient volitional airflow, continue to work on this horn in subsequent sessions.
    b. If the client is unable to blow the horn because he/she does not understand the concept of blowing to create a sound, return to either "Ah' in Supine or to "Bubble Blowing."
    c. If the client can blow the horn but is using a compensatory posture, inhibit that posture. Consultation with an occupational therapist or a physical therapist may be necessary if you are not familiar with these techniques. Once the posture is inhibited, instruct the client to blow that same horn again.
    d. If the client can blow the horn successfully at any number of repetitions but requires assisted jaw elevation or lip closure, continue to work on this horn in subsequent sessions until the assisted stability can be eliminated.
    e. <u>Criteria for Success:</u> If the client can blow the horn successfully 25 times in a row, without a break and without assisted jaw elevation or assisted lip closure, progress to the next horn on the hierarchy. As your skills improve in using horns for therapy, you will be able to estimate at which level you should begin the assessment component of therapeutic horn blowing.
5. Once you establish the highest level at which the client achieves success, right before failure, use that horn in Step #2.

## Step #2

1. The therapist places the tip of the mouthpiece on the client's lower lip as pictured previously. Instruct the client to blow the horn; monitor to ensure that no compensatory postures are being used (refer to 4. in Suggestions).
2. Remove and replace the horn after each repetition to re-establish the correct position in the mouth.

3. <u>Criteria for Success:</u> Have the client work up to blowing the targeted horn 25 times using the required time duration in repetitions, without a break, before progressing to the next horn on the hierarchy. Repeat this Step until all horns have been mastered.

**Note:** As your client progresses through the horn hierarchy, it will be the speech therapist's responsibility to transition these new skills in abdominal grading and jaw, lip and tongue placement into function for speech in each therapy session.

<u>Goals:</u>

1. Improve volitional airflow volume
2. Improve volitional airflow duration
3. Improve abdominal grading for increasing statement length
4. Reduce drooling
5. Improve jaw stability
6. Improve placement for labial and buccal control
7. Improve placement for lip closure and mentalis muscle control (Horns #1, 2, 3, 4, 5, 8)
8. Improve placement for lip rounding/protrusion (Horns #3, 6, 7, 9, 10)
9. Improve placement for tongue retraction and back of tongue side spread (Horn #9, 10, 11, 12)
10. Assist in jaw-lip-tongue dissociation to aid in improving co-articulation during conversational speech (improved speech clarity)
11. Teach awareness of articulator placement for individual target phoneme production (tactile-kinesthetic and proprioceptive feedback)
12. Improve motor planning through repetitive blowing (muscle memory).

<u>Target Phonemes:</u> All speech sounds

**Note:** *Horns as Therapy Tools*, by Sara Rosenfeld-Johnson, SLP, is a one-hour video designed to teach this OPT technique to therapists, parents, teachers, ect.

50

# GOLF BALL AIR HOCKEY

This activity is presented in the Phonation Section because it addresses deficits in abdominal grading and controlled oral airflow. It can also be used to improve articulation. A client who is using any speech sound error which is characterized by insufficient lip protrusion/lip rounding (i.e., tongue protrusion or tongue thrusting), and/or a too far forward tongue position can benefit from this technique. Remember, the harder the client blows, the greater the tongue retraction (lip protrusion results in tongue retraction).

The specific oral placement or movement goals are listed after each Step.

Suggestions:
1. This technique has been very successful with older clients who enjoy competition.
2. You will need a playing field, a ping pong ball, a "Whiffle" golf ball and a regular golf ball to implement this activity.
3. Prerequisite: Horn Blowing Hierarchy. Complete the Criteria for Success for Horn #8.
4. Homework: Establish during the session where the client fails on the hierarchy. Practice that Step at the highest level of successful repetitions for at least one week before moving on to the next level or Step.

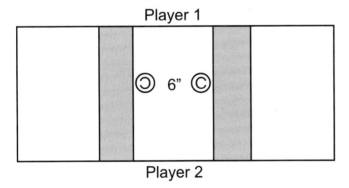
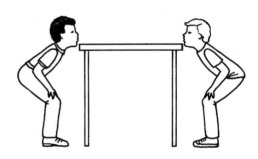

Step #1
1. Explain and establish the rules before you begin this game.

    Rules:
    a. The rules are similar to those used in hockey. A player receives one point for each successful goal.
    b. A goal is achieved when one player blows the ball over the other opponent's goal line or, in this case, over the edge of the table (refer to the picture above).

c. Each player's mouth must remain level with the table surface at all times, throughout the playing of a point.

d. The opponent receives one point when a penalty is observed. Penalties are given when the player:

    1) touches the ball with his/her mouth

    2) touches the table with his/her mouth for stability while blowing

    3) touches the table with his/her hands for support

e. A warning is given when the player puffs his/her cheeks out while blowing. The game is stopped and the ball is placed at the middle of the alley.

f. After each point is awarded, the ball is replaced at the middle of the alley.

g. Prior to each game, establish the criteria for winning the game based on the client's skill levels (10 to 21 points).

## Step #2

1. Set up the playing field (refer to the picture on the previous page).
2. Begin this activity with a ping-pong ball.
3. Place the ball at midpoint between the players, within the alley.
4. Instruct the opponents to work in a whispered "hoo" position (which will keep their cheeks tight) as they attempt to blow the ball over the other opponent's goal line.
5. Reward points as described above.
6. Criteria for Success: Ease of activity

Goals:

    1. Improve volitional airflow volume and duration

    2. Improve abdominal grading

    3. Improve endurance of orbicularis-oris muscle system for lip rounding

    4. Improve tongue retraction

    5. Maintain jaw-lip-tongue dissociation

## Target Phonemes:

1. Lip rounding/protrusion sounds: / w, o, u, ʊ, ɔ, ʃ(sh), ʧ(ch), ʤ(j) /

2. Tongue retraction sounds: all phonemes with the exception of /θ(th) and ð(th) /

3. The standard production of sibilants: / s, z, ʃ(sh), ʧ(ch), ʤ(j) /

## Step #3

1. Repeat Step #2 using a "Whiffle" golf ball.
2. Criteria for Success:  Ease of activity

Goals:

1. Improve volitional airflow volume and duration
2. Improve abdominal grading
3. Improve endurance of orbicularis-oris muscle system for lip rounding
4. Improve tongue retraction
5. Maintain jaw-lip-tongue dissociation

### Target Phonemes:

1. All lip rounding/protrusion sounds:  / w, o, u, ʊ, ɔ, ʃ(sh), ʧ(ch), ʤ(j) /

2. Tongue retraction sounds:  all phonemes with the exception of / θ(th) and ð(th) /

3. The standard production of sibilants:  / s, z, ʃ(sh), ʧ(ch), ʤ(j) /

## Step #4

1. Repeat Step #2 using a regular golf ball or a "magic eyeball."
2. Criteria for Success:  Ease of activity

Goals:

1. Improve volitional airflow volume and duration
2. Improve abdominal grading
3. Maintain tongue retraction
4. Maintain jaw-lip-tongue dissociation

### Target Phonemes:

a. All lip rounding/protrusion sounds:  / w, o, u, ʊ, ɔ, ʃ(sh), ʧ(ch), ʤ(j) /

b. Tongue retraction sounds: all phonemes with the exception of / θ(th) and ð(th) /

c. The standard production of sibilants: / s, z, ʃ(sh), ʧ(ch), ʤ(j) /

# ECHO HORN

Using an Echo Horn can be a fun visual way to teach the concept of phoneme imitation to the non-verbal child. Once the association is made between air from abdominal grading in combination with "something happening in the mouth" and sound production, molding that sound into phoneme imitation becomes more concrete. This technique is designed to associate phonation with exhalation (i.e., abdominal grading).

The specific oral placement or movement goals are listed after each Step.

Suggestions:

1. You will need an Echo Horn to implement this activity. Use a good quality Echo Horn as some of the cheaper versions do not echo loud enough.
2. The therapist/parent must hold the Echo Horn throughout this technique.
3. Hold the Echo Horn two to three inches from the client's mouth.
4. Because you will be working on improving oral placement or movement skills, a minimum of three repetitions is recommended.
5. This technique works well with the "Up-Up-Up Tickle" technique to associate controlled exhalation with phonation as a prerequisite for phoneme imitation.
6. Homework: Practice this technique with the parent and child working together for fun home reinforcement.

Step #1

1. Work in any position which will allow access to the abdominal muscles, as you may choose to place your palm on the abdominal muscles to associate exhalation with phonation.
   **Note:** Consultation with an occupational therapist or a physical therapist for position and movement suggestions is strongly recommended. Working on a large therapy ball has proven to be highly successful to assist in teaching the motor plan for volitional control of oral exhalations.
2. Hold the Echo Horn two to three inches from the client's mouth as the child is vocalizing, then immediately move the Echo Horn to your mouth and repeat the vocalization.
3. Return the Echo Horn to the client's mouth and wait for any vocalization.
   **Note:** If the client is unable to achieve volitional vocalization return to "Up-Up-Up Tickle," "Bubble Blowing" or "Horn Blowing" with transition to the kazoo to associate volitional exhalation with voiced phonation.

4. <u>Criteria for Success:</u> When 5 vocalizations are elicited in direct relationship to the Echo Horn placement, two to three inches from the client's mouth, progress to Step #2.

   <u>Goals:</u>

   1. Improve volitional airflow
   2. Increase the awareness that volitional exhalation is a prerequisite for vocalization
   3. Teach vocal turn taking as a prerequisite for phoneme imitation

<u>Step #2</u>

1. Choose single phonemes which have been used spontaneously in the client's vocal play.
2. Continue to alternate between your mouth and the client's mouth to teach the goal of phoneme imitation.

   **Note:** The Echo Horn changes and intensifies the auditory feedback, thereby increasing awareness. Use this technique to work on fine discrimination between standard phoneme productions and error sound productions.

3. <u>Criteria for Success:</u> Repeat until the client produces 5 different phoneme imitations consistently (e.g., you say "ah," then the client says "ah").

   <u>Goals:</u>

   1. Teach imitation of target phonemes
   2. Improve auditory discrimination between phoneme pairs

# MICROPHONE

Since not every client has the capacity for audible speech, it is sometimes important to give them the ability to be heard while you are working to improve their oral placement or movement skill levels. In this instance, you will be using a microphone to improve loudness for clients whose abdominal muscles cannot support their existing expressive language abilities within the classroom setting.

The specific oral placement or movement goals are listed after each Step.

Suggestions:

1. Continue to work on improving airflow duration and loudness through other activities.
2. When feasible, treatment with an occupational therapist/physical therapist is strongly suggested with these clients.
3. You will need a microphone with a volume control to implement this technique.

Step #1

1. Place the microphone 1 to 2 inches from the client's mouth.
2. Establish the lowest level at which the client can be heard clearly.
3. Position the microphone to be used functionally throughout the client's day.
4. Criteria for Success: Once acceptance/dependence of the microphone is established, progress to Step #2.

    Goals:

    1. Improve volitional oral airflow volume and duration
    2. Improve abdominal grading
    3. Improve loudness levels for functional communication
    4. Improve the client's ability to be heard by peers for increased socialization skill development

Step #2

1. Instruct the client to inhale through the mouth prior to speaking into the microphone.
2. Begin with vocalizations of only one syllable and expand to the number of syllables or words the client can produce on controlled exhalation. Monitor to ensure the client is not using compensatory "fixing."

    **Note:** Consultation with an occupational therapist or a physical therapist may be necessary if you are not familiar with compensatory posturing to increase airflow.

3. Refer to the activity called "Candle Blowing - Cake B" for further suggestions on teaching inhalation prior to vocalization.

4. Criteria for Success: Consistent audible usage of the microphone for interpersonal communication.

   Goal: Teach inhalation prior to speaking

## Step #3

1. Reduce the volume level on the microphone by one setting. Do this without the client's knowledge.

2. Position the microphone in the previously established location.

3. When the client speaks, indicate that he/she cannot be heard as well.

4. The client will automatically increase abdominal constriction/volitional airflow to accommodate the request for increased loudness.

5. Monitor to ensure compensatory body postures do not inhibit improved abdominal support.

6. Criteria for Success: Consistent audible usage of the microphone for interpersonal communication.

   Goals:

   1. Improve volitional oral airflow volume and duration
   2. Improve abdominal grading
   3. Increase loudness

## Step #4

1. Continue to reduce the volume level on the microphone in small increments every three to four weeks or as spontaneous loudness levels improve.

2. Criteria for Success: Eliminate dependence on the microphone when the client can be heard clearly without any amplification.

   Note: Exception: Some clients will never develop sufficient abdominal support, secondary to physiological deficits. These clients should be allowed to use microphones indefinitely.

   Goals:

   1. Improve volitional oral airflow and volume
   2. Increase loudness

# KAZOO

Use a kazoo to transition from silent oral airflow (e.g., horn blowing, bubble blowing, etc.) to vocalized oral airflow for improving speech clarity. For clients with motor-planning deficits, this may be a necessary step when moving from **PHONATION ACTIVITIES** to direct work on speech sound production. This technique is especially appropriate for clients with velopharyngeal insufficiency, secondary to structural or functional deficits.

The specific oral placement or movement goals are listed after each Step.

Suggestions:

1. Kazoos should not be included in a client's Program Plan when horn blowing is being used to develop abdominal grading. Once a client learns to vocalize while blowing, the effectiveness of the Horn Blowing Hierarchy will be compromised.

2. Prior to introducing a kazoo to assist in the transition from **PHONATION ACTIVITIES** to **RESONATION ACTIVITIES**, the following criteria will have to be met:
   a. "Horn Blowing Hierarchy" - Complete the Criteria for Success for Horn #8.
   b. "Bubble Blowing Hierarchy" - Complete the "Criteria for Success" for Step #4.

3. You will need two kazoos and two horns to implement this technique.

4. The therapist should hold the kazoo throughout this activity.

5. A small mirror can be placed under the nose to monitor any nasal airflow.

Step #1

1. Choose any horn the client can blow easily.

2. Criteria for Success: Work to 5 repetitions.

   Goal: Establish an oral airflow

Step #2

1. You will need two horns and two kazoos of the same style, one for each of you.

2. Holding one horn in your mouth and one horn in the client's mouth simultaneously, blow together 5 times.

3. Remove the horns and place the kazoo in your mouth. Vocalize an "oo" sound 5 times.

4. Place the same style kazoo in the client's mouth as you, simultaneously produce the "oo" sound with your kazoos.

58

**Note:** You may choose to keep the Kazoo in your mouth or to simply say the "oo" without the kazoo. Remember to reinforce any vocalization the client may make through the kazoo.

5. Criteria for Success: Once the client is able to produce the "oo" 5 times with the kazoo, without a break, progress to Step #3.

Goals:

1. Establish an oral airflow

2. Transition from silent airflow to an audible vocalization for speech

Step #3

1. Begin by allowing the client to make 5 "oo" sounds, using the kazoo, as you say "oo" without the kazoo.

2. Allow the client to use the kazoo to say "oo" 1 time, then remove it as you continue to say "oo" 4 more times.

3. By introducing and removing the kazoo from the client's mouth, encourage the repetition of "oo" with and without the kazoo.

4. Eliminate the use of the kazoo.

5. Criteria for Success: Repeat until the client is able to say "oo" 5 times in rapid succession, without the kazoo, using oral airflow.

Goals:

1. Transition from silent airflow to audible vocalization

2. Teach phoneme imitation

Step #4

1. Instruct the client to say "oo" 5 times without the kazoo. The kazoo will no longer be used for this activity.

2. Introduce "ah" as the next oral target phoneme. Work up to 5 oral imitations in rapid succession.

Goals:

1. Transition from silent airflow to audible vocalization

2. Teach phoneme imitation

Step #5

1. Introduce a variety of target phoneme imitations.

2. <u>Criteria for Success:</u> Repeat until the client is able to imitate 5 different target phonemes in rapid succession using oral airflow.

<u>Goals:</u>

1. Transition from silent airflow to audible vocalization
2. Teach phoneme imitation

# CHAPTER 5
# RESONATION ACTIVITIES

Before introducing any of the activities in this chapter, please make sure you have read the information in Chapters 1 and 2. The information given there is so important that it may be the difference between success and failure for you and for your client. Remember that maintaining a stable posture, throughout the completion of each Resonation Activity, will be required for maximum success during your therapy session, as well as during the implementation of homework assignments.

The techniques in this chapter are designed to improve velopharyngeal functioning as a component of speech clarity development. For normal resonation, we need both a supported nasal airflow and a supported oral airflow which can be redirected by the position of the velum. In many of our clients we have bypassed this critical muscle group, especially in the diagnosis of Down syndrome, Cerebral Palsy and severe Sensory-Neural Hearing Loss. In addition, we have negated the effectiveness of using blowing exercises (i.e., horn blowing, bubble blowing) as a technique for improving resonance in clients with a repaired cleft of the palate or velopharyngeal insufficiency.

We read over and over again, in our professional journals, that blowing does not improve oral airflow during speech sound production. For those of us who have worked in the field of speech therapy, we know this statement is true based on the existing research (i.e., research not performed on a hierarchy of blowing difficulty). The difference between traditional blowing therapy and the activities presented in this chapter is: **contrast**. The transition of oral airflow into vocalized oral airflow is then practiced in a vocalized oral-nasal contrast. By working in an oral-nasal contrast pattern, we are mobilizing the velum. Refer to the picture below as you imagine the velum is a person doing a sit-up. Pretend that blowing, using a vocalized oral airflow, is the person sitting up (a). If you continue to blow in this manner, the person's body does not have to move, therefore, no mobility is generated. Now pretend the use of the nasal phoneme / m / is made with the person lying down on the floor (b). Combine the two movements into an oral-nasal contrast (c). As you can see, repetitions of this activity will result in increasing mobility and control in the velum.

**(a)** 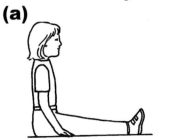   **(b)** 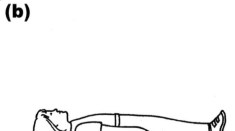   **(c)**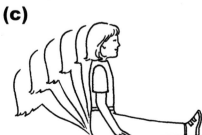

It is important to understand these techniques will not work for all clients. In many cases the structure is not sufficient to support normal velopharyngeal closure. If after two months of conscientious practice no progress is seen, you must refer the client to back to an ENT or cranio-facial team; other management may be indicated. If surgery is indicated, this activity program can then be re-introduced to mobilize the structure, after a surgical release has been obtained.

The activities presented in this chapter will be appropriate for clients who have any or all of the following goals:

1. Establish a controlled vocalized airflow
2. Establish a controlled vocalized nasal airflow
3. Establish oral-nasal contrast
4. Increase mobility in the velum
5. Improve velopharyngeal functioning
6. Use standard resonation: oral sounds and nasal sounds spontaneously at the conversational speech level
7. Teach nose blowing

**Note:** Each activity in this chapter will identify which of the goals outlined above you will be addressing.

# HUMMING #1

Humming can be used to establish volitional nasal airflow as a prerequisite for working on mobility of the velum through oral-nasal contrast work. It can also be used to establish volitional nasal airflow, when the client is healthy, as a prerequisite for teaching nose blowing.

The specific oral placement or movement goals are listed after each Step.

Suggestions:

1. Do not attempt this activity when the client is congested or has a documented nasal blockage.
2. Most children love music; Humming therefore, is frequently a favorite of even the most resistive of clients.
3. You will need a music source to implement this technique.
4. Homework: Establish during the session where the client fails on the hierarchy. Practice that Step at the highest level of successful repetitions for at least one week before moving onto the next level or Step.

Step #1

1. Use a tape or CD of the client's favorite music.
2. Begin with singing or vocalizing along with the music together with the client.
3. Cover your mouth and the client's mouth simultaneously but continue vocalizing. Change your vocalizations to humming.
   **Note:** If the client is unable to achieve this Step, return to a lower level off functioning (e.g., nasal exhalations to move a tissue, nasal exhalations to fog a mirror, nose flute).
4. Hum a favorite song in short beats of nasal air, approximately one second per beat.
5. Criteria for Success: Work up to 10 successful nasal beats before progressing to
   Goals:
   1. Establish a nasal airflow
   2. Stimulate movement of the velum as a prerequisite for improving velopharyngeal functioning

Step #2

1. Hum a favorite song using at least 10 short beats of nasal air.
2. Increase the length of the nasal exhalations in a breath group up to 4 seconds (1 unit).

63

3.  <u>Criteria for Success:</u>  Work up to 5 successive nasal breath group units.

<u>Goals:</u>

1. Establish a consistent nasal airflow

2. Improve mobility in the velum

3. Increase the volume and duration of volitional nasal airflow

# NOSE FLUTE

A nose flute can be used to establish volitional nasal airflow as a prerequisite for working on mobilizing the velum through oral-nasal contrast work. It can also be used to establish volitional nasal airflow as a means of helping to keep the client healthy. The ability to blow your nose when you are sick becomes a goal of therapy when you consider its benefits. When clients are unable to blow their nose, they are unable to clear the infection from their body; they stay sick longer. When they are sick, we cannot work with them to achieve our goals. If we can teach the client to effectively blow his/her nose, the client will get well sooner. We will then be able to work with that client more consistently. Learning to use a nose flute teaches the client a step-by-step technique to practice controlled nasal exhalation; it is a motor-planning tool for teaching nose blowing and achieving oral/nasal contrasts.

The specific oral placement or movement goals are listed after each Step.

Suggestions:

1. Do not attempt this activity when the client is congested or has a documented nasal blockage.
2. You will need a small rectangular mirror, a cotton ball or puff and two nose flutes to implement this technique.
3. Homework: Establish during the session where the client fails on the hierarchy.

Practice that Step at the highest level of successful repetitions for at least one week before moving onto the next level or Step.

Step #1

1. Place a small mirror under the client's nose, while holding the mouth closed, as pictured below.

   **Note:** Please do not attempt this technique unless the client trusts you.

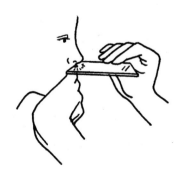

2. Talk about the "fog" that the nasal airflow has made on the surface of the mirror.
3. <u>Criteria for Success:</u>  Repeat 5 times before progressing to Step #2.

<u>Goals:</u>
1. Establish a nasal airflow
2. Stimulate movement of the velum as a prerequisite for improving velopharyngeal functioning

Step #2

1. Place the small mirror under the client's nose. Do not hold the mouth closed.
2. Instruct the client to "sniff" out to make the "fog" on the surface of the mirror bigger.
3. <u>Criteria for Success:</u>  Repeat 5 times before progressing to Step #3.

<u>Goal:</u>
1. Establish a stronger nasal airflow
2. Stimulate movement of the velum as a prerequisite for improving velopharyngeal functioning

Step #3

1. Place a light object (e.g., cotton ball or puff) on the surface of the mirror, closest to the child's nose, as pictured below.

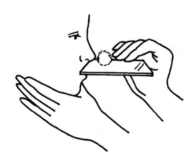

2. Instruct the client to "sniff" out to move the object over the edge of the mirror.
3. <u>Criteria for Success:</u>  Have the client "sniff" out to move the object 5 times over the edge of the mirror.

Step #4

1. Demonstrate the position and sound of the nose flute to the client using your own flute. Place the upper portion of the flute under your nose. Open your mouth and

place the lower portion inside your lower lip. Make sure there is a complete seal around your opened mouth and nose.

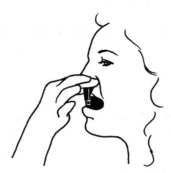

2. Exhale firmly through your nose. Call this production a "sniff."
3. Criteria for Success: Repeat 5 times.
   Goal: Demonstrate the use of the nose flute

Step #5
1. Place the client's nose flute on his/her face as described in Step #4.
2. Instruct the client to "sniff" firmly through the nose to elicit the sound.
3. <u>Criteria for Success:</u> Repeat this Step 10 times before progressing to Step #6.
   <u>Goals:</u>
   1. Establish a nasal airflow
   2. Stimulate movement of the velum as a prerequisite for improving velopharyngeal functioning

Step #6
1. Instruct the client to "sniff"/blow firmly through the nose flute to elicit the sound.
2. Work to elongate the sound of the nose flute by running your finger along the "Nasal Blow Path" as pictured.
3. Begin by running your finger quickly from "Start" to "Finish." As skill levels improve, slow down your movement to encourage prolongation of nasal airflow.
4. <u>Criteria for Success:</u> Prolong the sound of the nose flute for two seconds, 5 times.

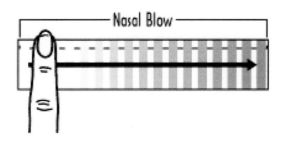

Goals:

1. Establish a consistent nasal airflow
2. Improve mobility in the velum
3. Increase the volume and duration of volitional nasal airflow

## Step #7

1. This Step will only be used when the client has mucous in the nasal cavity (e.g., when the client has a cold).
2. Place a tissue over the client's nose.
3. Instruct the client to pretend that he/she is "sniffing" out through the nose flute.

Goals:

1. Establish a consistent nasal airflow
2. Improve mobility in the velum
3. Increase the volume and duration of volitional nasal airflow
4. Teach nose blowing

# ORAL-NASAL CONTRASTS

This activity is used to normalize resonation by improving velopharyngeal functioning. Working on oral-nasal contrasts results in improved velopharyngeal closure and rate of movement, which directly affects standard production of oral phonemes and nasal phonemes in co-articulation.

The specific oral placement or movement goals are listed after each Step.

Suggestions:

1. Begin this activity when a consistent oral airflow has been established. Work through 25 repetitions of two seconds duration, without a break, using Horn #8 on the Horn Blowing Hierarchy before introducing this technique.

2. Begin this activity only when a consistent nasal airflow has been established. **Note:** If the client uses a habitual pattern of **hypernasality**, **assimilation nasality**, or **fluctuating nasality** (as observed in the low tone population), a consistent nasal airflow has been established.

3. If no nasal airflow is observed, a referral for a "medical causation evaluation" will be necessary, prior to introduction of this technique, to rule out nasal blockage.

4. After ruling out a nasal blockage, use the "Nose Flute" activity to establish a consistent nasal airflow, prior to the introduction of this technique.

5. You will need a Bubble Tube, a kazoo and 20 one-syllable items, pictures or written words to implement this activity.

6. As the difficulty of this technique increases, you will be increasing the length and complexity of the oral component while maintaining the isolated production of "m" as the nasal contrast.

7. Important: This technique may not work with all clients. If no progress is seen in any of the Steps after two months of conscientious practice, referral to back to an ENT or cranio-facial team is recommended. Other management may be indicated. A medical release should be obtained following any medical intervention prior to the initiation of oral placement therapy.

8. Homework: Establish during the session where the client fails on the hierarchy. Practice that Step at the highest level of successful repetitions for at least one week before moving onto the next level or Step.

Step #1

1. Use "Bubble Blowing" to establish oral airflow. Refer to the description of that activity if you have not used the technique prior to this contact.

2. Establish the whispered "hoo" position without supported jaw or lip stability.

3. Use a kazoo to transition from silent oral airflow to an audible vocalization of "hoo" (refer to the description of that technique in "Kazoo," if you have not used kazoos therapeutically prior to this contact).

4. Criteria for Success: Have the client work up to 10 totally oral repetitions of "hoo."
   Goals:
   1. Establish consistent oral airflow
   2. Establish consistent oral airflow for the production of "hoo"

Step #2

1. Begin with 10 oral repetitions of vocal "hoo." Use a small mirror placed under the nose to identify any nasal emissions.

2. Instruct the client to say "m" 10 times in rapid repetition.

3. Instruct the client to say "hoo" using a totally oral production, pause for one second, and then say "m" using tight lip closure for a totally nasal production. This step will establish the oral-nasal contrast.
   **Note**: The one-second pause, which will be the prescribed pause length throughout this activity, will allow for mobility and repositioning of the velum (i.e., - = one second pause).

4. Use the Oral-Nasal Contrast: "hoo" - (pause) "m" as 1 unit of repetition.

5. Criteria for Success: Work up to 10, 1-unit repetitions, without a break, before progressing to Step #3.
   Goals:
   1. Reinforce consistent oral airflow
   2. Stimulate movement of the velum as a prerequisite for improving velopharyngeal functioning

Step #3

1. Begin with 10 "hoo" - "m" contrasts.

2. Change the oral production while continuing to maintain the isolated production of the "m" as the nasal contrast:

"boo" - (pause) "m" = 10 times

"doo" - (pause) "m" = 10 times

"too" - (pause) "m" = 10 times

"poo" - (pause) "m" = 10 times

3. Criteria for Success:  Before progressing to Step #4, both voiced and unvoiced initial phonemes should be produced in the standard manner (10 repetitions in each category = 1 unit), 1 time.

**Note:** An exception would be made if voicing errors are consistent across articulation environments.  In such cases, using the error sounds would be acceptable.

Goals:

1. Reinforce consistent oral airflow

2. Improve velopharyngeal functioning

3. Stabilize oral airflow in a consonant-vowel production

Step # 4

1. Use any combination of oral consonants plus "oo" with the nasal contrast "m" in repetitions of 10 units, until it is obvious the skill has been mastered.

2. Create a string of 10 oral-nasal contrasts, using any combination you choose, maintaining the use of the vowel "oo" (10 contrasts = 1 unit).

Example:    "boo-m," "doo-m," "hoo-m," "foo-m," "soo-m," "koo-m," "goo-m," "poo-m," "loo-m," "roo-m"

3. Criteria for Success:  Have the client read or imitate the production of this string of contrasts (10 contrasts = 1 unit) in rapid succession 1 time, maintaining the integrity of the oral and the nasal production.

Goals:

1. Reinforce consistent oral airflow

2. Improve velopharyngeal functioning

3. Stabilize oral airflow in a string of consonant-vowel productions

Step #5

1. Generalize to other vowels and to consonant-vowel configurations in single contrasts.  Work at the one-syllable level.

Examples: "pie-m," "tuh-m," "fah-m"

71

2. Criteria for Success: Work up to strings of 10 oral-nasal contrasts (1 unit) one time, without a break, while maintaining the integrity of the oral-nasal production.

Goals:
1. Reinforce consistent oral airflow
2. Improve velopharyngeal functioning
3. Stabilize oral airflow in a string of varying consonant-vowel productions

Step #6
1. Establish a list of 20 one-syllable words having only oral phonemes. For younger children use single-syllable items on picture cards.
2. Present the words or pictures as oral nasal contrasts:
   Examples: "boy-m," "car-m," "hat-m," "sit-m," "fox-m," etc.
3. Criteria for Success: Work up to 20 words (1 unit), 1 time, while maintaining the integrity of the oral-nasal contrast.

Goals:
1. Reinforce consistent oral airflow
2. Improve velopharyngeal functioning
3. Stabilize oral airflow on the single-word level

Step #7
1. Use a 4" x 6" index card with the word "The" followed by _____ - "m."

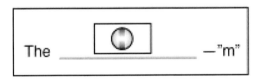

2. Place the picture cards used in Step #6, one at a time, on the line to stimulate the production of "The + (word) - m."
3. Criteria for Success: Require the client to produce all 20 words in the above described phrase, without a break, while maintaining the integrity of the oral-nasal contrast.

Goals:
1. Reinforce consistent oral airflow
2. Improve velopharyngeal functioning
3. Expand oral airflow to a two-word production

## Step #8

1. Use a 4" x 6" index card with the word "The" followed by ____ is - " m."

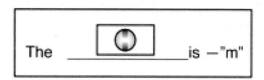

2. Place the picture cards used in Steps #6 and #7, one at a time, on the line to stimulate the production of: "The + (word) is - m."
3. <u>Criteria for Success:</u>  Require the client to produce all 20 words in the above-described phrase (1 unit) 1 time, without a break, while maintaining the integrity of the oral-nasal contrast.

   <u>Goals:</u>
   1. Reinforce consistent oral airflow
   2. Improve velopharyngeal functioning
   3. Expand oral airflow to a three-word production

## Step #9

1. Continue to increase, in one-syllable increments, the length of the oral component of the oral-nasal contrast.

   **Note:** Whenever there is a nasalized production of an oral sound or an oralized production of a nasal sound, bring the error to the client's attention and return to a lower level on the hierarchy.

2. <u>Criteria for Success:</u> Continue until carryover into conversational speech is noted.

   <u>Goals:</u>
   1. Reinforce consistent oral airflow
   2. Improve velopharyngeal function
   3. Use standard resonation: oral sounds and nasal sounds spontaneously on the conversational speech level

## SINGING-HUMMING

This activity is used to normalize resonation by improving velopharyngeal functioning. Working on oral-nasal contrasts (singing-humming) results in improved velopharyngeal closure and rate of movement, which directly affects standard production of oral phonemes in co-articulation.

The specific oral placement or movement goals are listed after each Step.

Suggestions:
1. Do not begin this technique until the client has successfully completed Step #8 in the "Oral-Nasal Contrast" activity.
2. Begin this technique when the client has successfully completed Step #1 in the "Humming" activity.

Step #1
1. Review "Humming" to establish that the client is able to maintain a nasal airflow while vocalizing.
2. Use the chart below. Put your pointer finger in the ☐ box when you want the client to sing "oo" and in the ■ box when you want the client to hum "m" (1 unit).

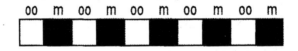

3. <u>Criteria for Success:</u> Repeat this unit 5 times as you move from box ☐ to box ■.

Step #2
1. Use the chart below and a familiar song to introduce the concept of alternating singing with humming.
2. Establish a pattern of 1 beat per box, as you work down the path from the beginning to the end. If the song is longer than the path, return to the beginning and work toward the end.

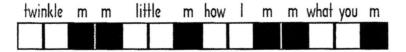

3. <u>Criteria for Success:</u> Continue until an entire familiar song can be sung and hummed, using the above contrast chart, while maintaining the integrity of the oral or the nasal production.

<u>Goals:</u>

1. Reinforce consistent oral airflow
2. Reinforce consistent nasal airflow
3. Improve velopharyngeal-pharyngeal functioning

# CHAPTER 6
# ARTICULATION ACTIVITIES

Before using any of the suggestions in this chapter, please make sure you have read the information in Chapters 1 and 2. The information given there is so important that it may be the difference between success and failure for you and for your client. Remember, that maintaining a stable body posture, throughout the completion of each **Articulation Activity**, will be required for maximum success during your therapy session, as well as during the implementation of homework assignments.

The techniques in this chapter are divided into three sections:

**SECTION 1 - JAW ACTIVITIES**
**SECTION 2 - LIP ACTIVITIES**
**SECTION 3 - TONGUE ACTIVITIES**

Refer to the in-depth description in Chapter 3 of how and when to use the various activities in these sections.

## SECTION 1 - JAW ACTIVITIES

Jaw activities will be used for clients who have any or all of the following goals:

1. Teach an optimal or natural bite posture
2. Improve jaw alignment
3. Improve jaw stability
4. Improve jaw grading and dissociation
5. Establish stability in the jaw as a prerequisite for the development of standard co-articulation of all speech sounds

**Note:** Remember, many of the activities presented earlier, in the chapters entitled **"Phonation"** and **"Resonation,"** are also working on jaw stability and grading.

## SECTION 2 - LIP ACTIVITIES

Lip activities will be used for clients who have any or all of the following goals:

1. Improve awareness of the lips as a prerequisite for improving speech sound production
2. Reduce/eliminate drooling
3. Teach lip closure for speech sound production of bi-labial speech sounds
4. Teach lip rounding for speech sound production of lip rounding sounds

5. Teach lip retraction for speech sound production of lip retraction sounds

6. Teach lower lip retraction for speech sound production /f/ and /v/ sounds

7. Teach lower lip protrusion for speech sound production of ʃ(sh), tʃ(ch), ʤ(j), /r/ and the vocalic /r/

8. Develop jaw-lip dissociation for improved speech clarity on the level of co-articulation

   **Note:** Remember, many of the activities presented earlier, in the chapters entitled **"Phonation"** and **"Resonation,"** are also working on lip closure, rounding, protrusion and/or retraction.

## SECTION 3 - TONGUE ACTIVITIES

Tongue activities will be used for clients who have any or all of the following goals:

1. Teach tongue retraction for speech sound production of all phonemes made within the oral cavity (i.e., all sounds in English with the exception of the voiced and voiceless "th")

2. Teach tongue-tip lateralization as a prerequisite for tongue-tip elevation

3. Teach tongue-tip elevation for speech sound production of tongue-tip elevation sounds

4. Teach tongue-tip depression for speech sound production of tongue-tip depression sounds

5. Teach back of tongue side spread for isolated speech sound production and co-articulation

6. Develop jaw-lip-tongue dissociation as a prerequisite for the development of standard co-articulation of all speech sounds on the conversational level

   **Note:** Remember, many of the activities presented earlier, in the chapters entitled **"Phonation," "Resonation"** and **"Articulation,"** are also working on tongue retraction, tongue-tip elevation, tongue-tip depression and back of tongue side spread.

77

# SECTION 1 - JAW ACTIVITIES

Historically, when we have looked at and listened to a client who has a speech clarity disorder, we rarely noticed what the jaw was doing. Instead, we concentrated on how the lips and tongue were moving. The jaw is the most neglected component of an articulation skill evaluation. Lip placement and tongue placement are secondary to jaw position. For standard production of each speech sound, the jaw must maintain proper height and position while allowing the lips and tongue to move independently. Jaw jutting or sliding will directly impact on the clarity of what is being said. If the jaw is not strong enough to support dissociated lip and tongue movements, intelligibility will be reduced significantly.

**Symmetrical strength** and **stability,** in the muscles of the jaw, are necessary for **jaw grading** to develop. Without jaw grading, speech sound production will be distorted. In order to understand jaw grading, refer to Picture #1 and the Consonant and Vowel Chart below:

Picture #1

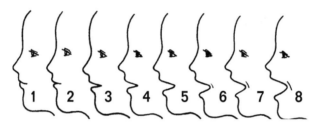

Consonant and Vowel Chart

|  | | Consonants | Vowels | |
|---|---|---|---|---|
| Jaw Height | High | m b p f v n s z ʃ tʃ r | I e u v | Closed ↓ Open |
| | Medium | θ ʒ l  td | ʌ o ɔ ɛ | |
| | Low | g k h | æ a | |

Place your thumb under your chin. Make sure your arm is not resting on a table, etc. The presence of your thumb is to allow you to feel what happens to your jaw when you say isolated speech sounds. Therefore, allow your thumb to follow your jaw, not to direct it. It is even more valuable if you are able to feel the proprioceptive and **kinesthetic feedback** from the movement of the jaw during phoneme production. As you say each sound, notice that your jaw elevates or depresses. Try to say a / m / with your jaw in a **low jaw posture** without moving the jaw. It is impossible.

Many of our clients do not have adequate jaw grading necessary to support co-articulation. Instead, they utilize either a **high jaw fixed posture** or a **low jaw fixed posture** to compensate for this lack of grading. Position your jaw as pictured below. Try to speak without moving your jaw. Speech clarity is significantly reduced when the jaw does not grade.

**High Jaw Fixed Posture**

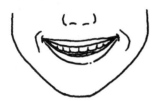

**Low Jaw Fixed Posture**

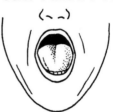

Jaw sliding during speech sound production is generally noted secondary to symmetrical jaw instability/weakness. Jutting of the jaw, during speech sound production, may be secondary to: (1) Asymmetrical jaw instability/weakness or (2) Non-dissociation of the tongue from the jaw (the tongue pushing on the lower jaw in association with the production of a specific sound or a group of sounds). It will be important to diagnosis the reason for the jaw slide or jut prior to initiating a treatment protocol as the number of repetitions per side will depend on the diagnostic information.

Jaw instability is the most common cause for deterioration of speech clarity when the speed or complexity of an utterance increases. When you write the sentence, "As the rate of speech increases, the intelligibility decreases," you are frequently describing that the client's jaw is not stable enough to allow for dissociated movements of the lips and tongue. When the jaw is not stable, the lips and the tongue cannot do their job for standard speech production.

Remember, one of the best ways to improve jaw stability is to teach the client to chew on the back molars.

# TALKTOOLS® JAW GRADING BITE BLOCKS:

## Assessment and Treatment Protocol

This assessment and treatment protocol, which follows the Chewy Tube™ and ARK's Grabber Assessment and Treatment Protocols, can be used with both children and adults. In this exercise, the TalkTools® Jaw Grading Bite Blocks are first used to assess jaw skill levels, and then to work toward improving jaw strength, symmetry and grading. The skills acquired in this exercise can then be transitioned into improved feeding safety and the graded movements necessary for standard speech sound production on the single sound and conversational levels. This exercise requires that the client be able to follow the verbal command of "bite and hold."

## <u>Natural Bite:</u>

Prior to their introduction to the TalkTools® Jaw Grading Bite Block Exercises, the client must demonstrate the ability to bite down on Bite Block #2, using their natural bite, on both sides of the mouth. Use the following exercise for assessment and treatment of a natural bite posture.

<u>Suggestions:</u>

1. You will need a cubed solid and two Bite Blocks #2 to implement this prerequisite task.

2. Before introducing any food items, a complete feeding history (including dietary limitations, possible food allergies and list of safe food textures and preferences) must be compiled.

3. If you observe a jaw jut but are unable to determine if it is structural or functional, referral to a dentist or orthodontist will be necessary.

4. The client does not have to be able to follow verbal directions to benefit from this exercise.

5. The client's head must be maintained at midline as the task is being practiced.

6. Using a mirror may be helpful for some clients who need visual reinforcement in addition to kinesthetic feedback. For other clients the presence of a mirror may be confusing (as the visual image is reversed) or distracting.

7. Use the TalkTools® Jaw Grading Bite Block Assessment and Treatment Form on page 98 to record diagnostic information and chart progress.

8. Homework: Establish during the session where the client fails on the hierarchy of difficulty. Practice that step at the highest level of repetitions, 1-3 times per day at a minimum of 3 times per week or until that step is mastered.

80

9. <u>Criteria for Success:</u> The criteria for success is listed after each step in the task. Once the client has mastered the criteria for one step, you are free to introduce the next. If the client does not achieve the criteria for success, continue to practice that step until they can do so before progressing to the next step on the hierarchy.

<u>Step #1</u>

1. Instruct the client to close his/her teeth while keeping the lips open. Observe the bite alignment.
2. Place a single cubed solid on the surface of the left side lower back molars. Instruct the client to chew as you observe the bite-chew alignment.
3. Repeat on the right side of the mouth and observe the bite-chew alignment.
4. Place Bite Block #2 on the surface of the left side lower back molars extending from the front of the mouth, as pictured below. Instruct the client to bite down on the Bite Block.
   **Note:** the alignment, then remove the Bite Block.

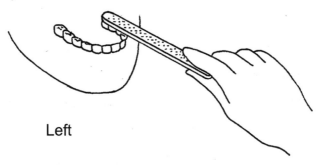

Left

5. Place Bite Block #2 on the surface of the right side lower back molars extending from the front of the mouth, as pictured below. Instruct the client to bite down on the Bite Block.
   **Note:** the alignment and remove the Bite Block.

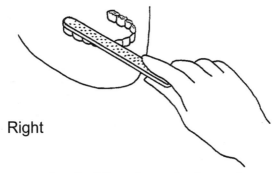

Right

6. If the alignment is the same in all of the above tasks and you do not see any jaw jutting, you are probably observing the client's natural bite. Enter the information on the blank TalkTools® Jaw Grading Bite Block Assessment and Treatment Form on page 98, then begin with the Bite Block exercises on page 91.

7. If there is inconsistency in the jaw alignment in any of the above tasks, proceed to Step #2 of this exercise to teach a natural bite.
8. <u>Criteria for Success:</u> The client demonstrates the same bite position in each of the following situations: (a) biting down with lips open, (b) biting and chewing on a cubed solid on both sides of the mouth, and (c) biting down on Bite Block #2 on both sides of the mouth.

<u>Step #2</u>

1. Place your fingertips on the client's temporomandibular joint as you use the heel of both hands to support the chin. Do not press or push too firmly. Use your hands to feel the alignment of the jaw as it opens and closes.
2. Instruct the client to bite down. Feel if the jaw juts forward or to either side as the client bites down.
3. Instruct the client to bite down using the natural bite. Repeat this task 5 times.
4. If the jaw does not move out of alignment, progress to Step #3. If the jaw moves out of alignment, continue to teach the natural bite by repeating the task described in this step.

   **Note:** If the client with whom you are working cannot understand the verbal direction, or visual model, try a tactile cue. Place your index finger under the mandible, just off the bony process. Gently push upward on the jaw to facilitate a natural bite.
5. <u>Criteria for Success:</u> The client is able to bite down without any evidence of jaw jutting or sliding while the therapist uses both hands to support the jaw, 5 times.

<u>Step #3</u>

1. Place one Bite Block #2 on the surface of the left side lower back molars, extending from the side of the mouth, and one Bite Block #2 on the surface of the right side molars, also extending from the side of the mouth, as pictured below. Instruct the client to bite down.

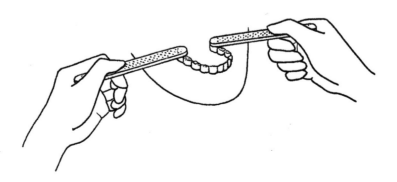

2. Instruct the client to bite down using the natural bite. Repeat this task 5 times.
3. If the jaw does not move out of alignment, progress to Step #4. If it does move out of alignment, continue to teach the natural bite by repeating the task described in this step.
4. <u>Criteria for Success:</u> The client is able to bite down on two Bite Blocks #2, without any evidence of jaw jutting or sliding, 5 times.

## Step #4

1. Place one Bite Block #2 on the surface of the left side lower back molars, extending from the side of the mouth, and one Bite Block #2 on the right side surface, also extending from the side of the mouth, as pictured below. Instruct the client to bite down.

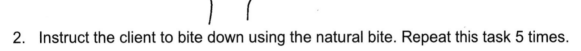

2. Instruct the client to bite down using the natural bite. Repeat this task 5 times.
3. If the jaw does not move out of alignment, progress to Step #5. If it does move out of alignment, continue to teach the natural bite by repeating the task described in this step.
4. <u>Criteria for Success:</u> The client is able to bite down on two Bite Blocks #2, without any evidence of jaw jutting or sliding, 5 times.

## Step #5

1. Place one Bite Block #2 on the surface of the left lower back molars, extending from the front of the mouth, and one Bite Block #2 on the right side surface, also extending from the front of the mouth, as pictured below. Instruct the client to bite down.

83

2.  Instruct the client to bite down using the natural bite. Repeat this task 5 times.

3.  If the jaw does not move out of alignment, progress to Step #6. If it does move out of alignment, continue to teach the natural bite by repeating the task described in this step.

4.  Criteria for Success: The client is able to bite down on two Bite Blocks #2, without any evidence of jaw jutting or sliding, 5 times.

Step #6

1.  Instruct the client to bite down using their natural bite, without using the Bite Blocks. Repeat this task 5 times.

2.  If the jaw does not move out of alignment, progress to the TalkTools® Jaw Grading Bite Block Exercises on page 91.

3.  If the jaw moves out of alignment, continue to teach the natural bite by repeating the task described in this step.

4.  Criteria for Success: The client is able to bite down using his/her natural bite, without the benefit of any therapy tool, 10 times.

# TALKTOOLS® JAW GRADING BITE BLOCK EXERCISES

**Assessment and Treatment (Jaw Height Levels #2 - #7)**

This exercise is designed to teach symmetrical jaw strength at each jaw height position as a component of developing jaw stability, dissociation and grading, all of which are prerequisites for the development of independent lip and tongue movements and standard co-articulation of all speech sounds. The tools are first used to diagnose jaw stability or instability, and are then used for exercise to create jaw stability.

Suggestions:

1. You will need two sets of TalkTools® Jaw Grading Bite Blocks or TalkTools® Sensory Friendly Jaw Grading Bite Blocks to implement all of the Bite Block Exercises. None of these tools require more strength in the jaw than is necessary for safe feeding or standard speech sound production.

2. Prior to introducing this exercise the client must be able to demonstrate two controlled, natural bites on the green ARK's Grabber, as detailed in the ARK's Grabbers Assessment and Treatment Protocol Exercise.

3. The jaw assessment and treatment protocol must be performed in the natural bite position. Working in a jaw slide or jaw jut position is a compensatory posture and therefore will not achieve the targeted goals. Directions for identifying if the client is using his/her natural bite can be found beginning on page 80.

4. If the client does not have the cognitive ability or motor skills necessary to follow the directions for the Prerequisite - Bite and Hold Exercise, you will not be able to use any of the TalkTools® Jaw Grading Bite Block Exercises. Instead, use the exercises that are stimulus-response based (i.e., ARK's Probe, ARK's Z-Vibe, Chewy Tubes, ARK's Grabbers, Firm Licorice Stick, Slow Feed, Cube Placement and the Gum Chewing Program).

5. As part of the assessment you will need to determine if the weakness in the jaw musculature is symmetrical or asymmetrical. Speech is characterized by symmetrical jaw strength which is sufficient to support jaw grading and dissociated lip and tongue movements.

6. There are three exercises at each Bite Block level. The Bite Blocks are numbered according to jaw height. Therefore, there is no #1 Bite Block, as this jaw height would be achieved with the teeth closed in a natural bite posture. No standard speech sounds are made at Jaw Height Level #1. The Bite Blocks are numbered 2 through 7, representing Jaw Heights #2 through #7 on the chart below, as these heights are used in standard speech production

85

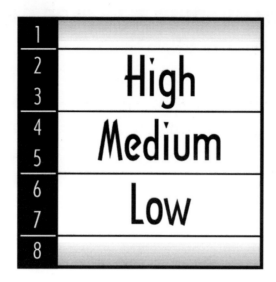

7. The client's head must be maintained at midline during both the assessment and treatment phases of this exercise.
8. In most cases you will begin with Bite Block #2 and work through the hierarchy to Bite Block #7. Maximum results for these clients will be achieved if this exercise is practiced in conjunction with the Slow Feed Exercise and the Gum Chewing Program.
9. For clients who are unable to bite down on Bite Block #2, secondary to high tone (i.e., cerebral palsy, traumatic brain injury, etc.), begin with Bite Block #7 and work to Bite Block #2. For these clients you will not be able to use the Slow Feed Exercise or the Gum Chewing Program as these exercises at Jaw Height #7 would place them at high risk for choking and gagging.
10. The assessment is complete when the client either achieves the criteria for success for all three exercises using the TalkTools® Jaw Grading Bite Blocks #2 - #7 or fails to meet the required criteria at any level on any of the three exercises. You will begin your exercises, in therapy and at home, at the highest level before failure.
11. The following four exercises are presented in a hierarchy. You will complete them in the following order, both in the assessment and in therapy:

Prerequisite – Bite and Hold

Exercise A - Bite Block

Exercise B - Twin Bite Blocks for Symmetrical Jaw Stability

Exercise C - Bite Block for Jaw Stability

12. If the client is pulled forward as you are using the isometric pull, consider the following possibilities:
    a. You may be pulling too hard. In this case, use less resistance.
    b. You may be working at too high a level. In this case, return to a lower level.
    c. The behavior may be habitual rather than functional. In this case, use a therapy pillow as a tactile cue.

13. In order to avoid injury to the jaw, the following principles must be acknowledged in each of the exercises:
    a. Monitor to ensure that the client is not using whole body compensatory postures to pull back on the Bite Blocks; the resistance should be localized to the jaw musculature.
    b. If the client uses excessive force in the jaw, the temporomandibular joint may be injured.
    c. The client should only be biting hard enough to keep the Bite Block from being pulled out of his/her mouth.
    d. Do not work beyond the prescribed number of repetitions.

14. In this exercise you will both diagnose and treat jaw skill deficits. Use the blank TalkTools® Jaw Grading Bite Block Assessment and Treatment Form, which can be found on page 98, to record your data and note progress.

15. Once your client has completed the diagnostic workup, refer to the section labeled Using the Correct Diagnostic Term, on page 99, prior to initiating your therapeutic intervention.

16. If at any time during the practice of this exercise the client appears to be seeking additional sensory information, the tip of the Bite Block can be dipped in ice water, sensory powder, extract or a highly-flavored liquid to increase awareness and/or acceptance. Please note that before introducing any food items a complete feeding history, including dietary limitations, possible food allergies and a list of safe food textures and preferences, must be compiled.

17. This exercise is frequently used in conjunction with the Chewy Tube™ Exercises, ARK's Grabber Exercises, ARK's Z-Vibe, Firm Licorice Stick, Slow Feed, Cube Placement and the Gum Chewing Program as a component of program plans designed to treat jaw weakness or instability.

18. This exercise should be performed in a stable seating posture as described earlier in this chapter on page 86.

87

19. Isometric resistance therapy is used to improve strength in a muscle or muscle group; pulling on the muscle so hard that it goes out of alignment is not recommended or necessary. When using isometric resistance use only a gentle pull. Your goal is to give slight resistance to stimulate a slightly stronger bite, not to injure the temporomandibular joint.

20. Homework: Establish during the session where the client fails on the hierarchy of instructions. Practice that step at the highest level of repetitions 1-3 times per day for a minimum of 3 times per week or until that step has been mastered.

21. Criteria for Success: The criteria for success is listed after each step in the exercise. Once the client has mastered the criteria for success for one step, you are free to move on to the next. If the client does not achieve the criteria for success, continue to practice at that step until the criteria for success have been met before progressing to the next step on the hierarchy.

# ASSESSMENT - Assessment Procedure (Diagnostic)

## PREREQUISITE – BITE AND HOLD:

You must first establish that the client can bite and hold the Bite Block, in a natural bite position and without moving the jaw, before progressing to the diagnostic component of the TalkTools® Jaw Grading Bite Block Exercises.

### Step #1

1. Place the tip of Bite Block #2 on the surface of the left lower back molars, extending from the front of the mouth as pictured below. Instruct the client to use a natural bite posture to bite down on the Bite Block.

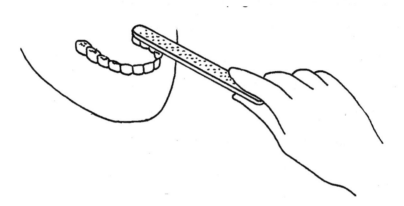

   **Note**: A natural bite is defined as the optimal bite alignment that can be achieved with the existing jaw and dental structures. For further information concerning a natural bite posture, refer to the Natural Bite Exercise on page 80.

2. Instruct the client to continue to bite without moving the jaw, thereby maintaining the natural bite posture. Hold this bite for 3 seconds, 1 time.

   **Note**: If the client opens his/her mouth, or moves the jaw even slightly, you must remove the Bite Block and repeat the task.

3. Repeat on the right side of the mouth.

4. <u>Criteria for Success</u>: With the #2 Bite Block in place, hold the natural bite posture for 3 seconds without any evidence of jaw or head movement, on alternating sides of the mouth, 1 time.

### Step #2

1. Place the tip of the #2 Bite Block on the surface of the left lower back molars, extending from the front of the mouth as described above. Instruct the client to use a natural bite posture to bite down on the Bite Block.

2. Instruct the client to continue to bite without moving the jaw, thereby maintaining the natural bite posture. Hold this bite for 4 seconds, 1 time.

   **Note:** If the client opens his/her mouth, or moves the jaw even slightly, you must remove the Bite Block and repeat the task.

3. Repeat on the right side of the mouth.

4. Criteria for Success: With the #2 Bite Block in place, hold the natural bite posture for 4 seconds without any evidence of jaw or head movement, on alternating sides of the mouth, 1 time.

## Step #3

1. Repeat the Bite and Hold technique as described in Step #2, increasing the duration of the "hold" segment in 1-second increments until a 10-second hold is achieved on both the left and right sides of the mouth, 1 time.

   **Note:** If the client opens his/her mouth, or moves the jaw even slightly, you must remove the Bite Block and repeat the task.

2. Criteria for Success: With the #2 Bite Block in place, hold the natural bite posture for 10 seconds without any evidence of jaw or head movement, on alternating sides of the mouth, 1 time.

## Step #4

1. Now that the client has met the criteria for success on both sides of the mouth, enter that information on the TalkTools® Jaw Grading Bite Block Assessment and Treatment Form as pictured below. A blank copy of this form can be found on page 98.

## TalkTools® Jaw Grading Bite Block Assessment and Treatment Form

| Tool | A. Bite Block Exercise | B. Twin Bite Block for Symmetrical Jaw Stability Exercise | C. Bite Block for Jaw Stability Exercise |
|---|---|---|---|
| Prerequsite Bite and Hold | ✓ 10 sec. R ✓ 10 sec L (1X) | | |

Proceed to the exercise entitled **Exercise A - Bite Block.**

90

# EXERCISE A – BITE BLOCK

<u>Step #1</u>

1. Place the tip of the #2 Bite Block on the surface of the left lower back molars, extending from the front of the mouth as pictured below. Instruct the client to use a natural bite posture to bite down on the Bite Block.

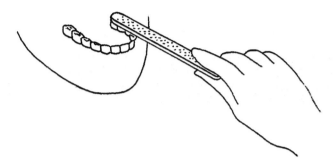

2. Explain to the client that you are going to pull the Bite Block forward (toward you) using an isometric pull. You will only be using a small amount of resistance.
   **Note**: An isometric pull is defined as a pull that is strong enough to make the client work only slightly harder to keep the Bite Block from being pulled out of the mouth. It is not so hard as to require the client to bite down with such tension that you see a bulge in the cheek muscles.
3. While maintaining the natural bite posture, pull forward using isometric resistance until you reach the goal of 15 seconds or the client fails to achieve the 15-second goal.
   **Note:** Failure is described as seen in any of the following scenarios:
   a. The client cannot maintain their hold on the Bite Block and it comes out of the mouth.
   b. The client uses any of the following compensatory postures to keep the Bite Block in his/her mouth: moves forward, moves backward, turns the head, uses whole body tension to maintain the bite on the therapy tool, or uses hands to hold the jaw closed.
4. Make a note of the 15-second success on the left side or the number of seconds achieved before failure.
5. Repeat on the right side of the mouth.
6. <u>Criteria for Success:</u> Hold the natural bite posture on the #2 Bite Block for 15 seconds while maintaining the isometric pull, on first the left and then the right side of the mouth, without any evidence of compensatory patterns, 1 time.

Step #2   One of the following scenarios will be evident:

1.   If the client can meet the criteria for success on both sides of the mouth, place two check marks in the chart below, as indicated, and proceed to the next exercise in the sequence, **Exercise B - Twin Bite Blocks for Symmetrical Jaw Stability** on page 93.

### TalkTools® Jaw Grading Bite Block Assessment and Treatment Form

| Tool | A. Bite Block Exercise | B. Twin Bite Block for Symmetrical Jaw Stability Exercise | C. Bite Block for Jaw Stability Exercise |
|---|---|---|---|
| Prerequsite Bite and Hold | _✓_ 10 sec. R _✓_ 10 sec L (1X) | | |
| Bite Block #2 | _✓_ 15 sec. R _✓_ 15 sec L (1X) | _____15 sec. R & L (1X) | _____15 sec. (1X) |

2.   If the client cannot meet the 15-second criteria for success on one or both sides of the mouth, enter the highest number achieved before failure in the chart below as indicated in the following example. Your assessment is now complete. Proceed to Using the Correct Diagnostic Term on page 99.

### TalkTools® Jaw Grading Bite Block Assessment and Treatment Form

| Tool | A. Bite Block Exercise | B. Twin Bite Block for Symmetrical Jaw Stability Exercise | C. Bite Block for Jaw Stability Exercise |
|---|---|---|---|
| Prerequsite Bite and Hold | _✓_ 10 sec. R _✓_ 10 sec L (1X) | | |
| Bite Block #2 | _12_ 15 sec. R _12_ 15 sec L (1X) | _____15 sec. R & L (1X) | _____15 sec. (1X) |

# EXERCISE B – TWIN BITE BLOCKS FOR SYMMETRICAL JAW STABILITY

Step #1

1. Place the tip of a #2 Bite Block on the surface of the lower back molars on both sides of the mouth, extending from the front of the mouth as pictured below. Instruct the client to bite down on the Bite Blocks using a natural bite posture.

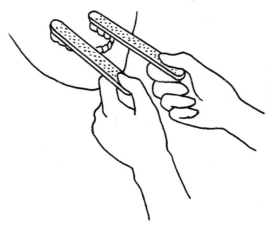

2. Explain to the client that you are going to pull the Bite Blocks forward (toward you) using an isometric pull. You will only be using a small amount of resistance.

   **Note:** An isometric pull is defined as a pull that is strong enough to make the client work only slightly harder to keep the Bite Blocks from being pulled out of the mouth. It is not so hard as to require the client to bite down with such tension that you see a bulge in the cheek muscles.

3. While maintaining the natural bite posture, pull forward using isometric resistance until you reach the goal of 15 seconds or the client fails to achieve the 15-second goal.

   **Note:** Failure is described as seen in any of the following scenarios:

   a. The client cannot maintain the hold on the Bite Blocks and one or both come out of the mouth.

   b. The client uses any of the following compensatory postures to keep the Bite Blocks in his/her mouth: moves forward, moves backward, turns the head, uses whole body tension to maintain the bite on the therapy tools, or uses hands to hold the jaw closed.

4. Make a note of the 15-second success or the number of seconds achieved before failure.

5. Criteria for Success: Hold the natural bite posture on the #2 Twin Bite Blocks for 15 seconds while maintaining the isometric pull, without any evidence of compensatory patterns, 1 time.

<u>Step #2</u>   One of the following scenarios will be evident:

1.  If the client can meet the criteria for success, place a check mark in the chart below as indicated and proceed to the next exercise in the sequence, **Exercise C - Bite Block for Jaw Stability** page 95.

**TalkTools® Jaw Grading Bite Block Assessment and Treatment Form**

| Tool | A. Bite Block Exercise | B. Twin Bite Block for Symmetrical Jaw Stability Exercise | C. Bite Block for Jaw Stability Exercise |
|---|---|---|---|
| Prerequsite Bite and Hold | _✓_ 10 sec. R _✓_ 10 sec L (1X) | | |
| Bite Block #2 | _✓_ 15 sec. R _✓_ 15 sec L (1X) | _✓_15 sec. R & L (1X) | _____15 sec. (1X) |

2.  If the client cannot meet the 15-second criteria for success, enter the highest number achieved before failure in the chart below as indicated in the example. Your assessment is now complete. Proceed to Using the Correct Diagnostic Term on page 99.

**TalkTools® Jaw Grading Bite Block Assessment and Treatment Form**

| Tool | A. Bite Block Exercise | B. Twin Bite Block for Symmetrical Jaw Stability Exercise | C. Bite Block for Jaw Stability Exercise |
|---|---|---|---|
| Prerequsite Bite and Hold | _✓_ 10 sec. R _✓_ 10 sec L (1X) | | |
| Bite Block #2 | _✓_ 15 sec. R _✓_ 15 sec L (1X) | _14_ 15 sec. R & L (1X) | _____15 sec. (1X) |

# EXERCISE C – BITE BLOCK FOR JAW STABILITY

Step #1

1. Place a single #2 Bite Block on the surface of the lower teeth horizontally, extending from the sides of the mouth as pictured below. Instruct the client to use a natural bite posture to bite down on the Bite Block.

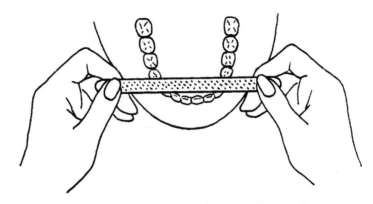

2. Explain to the client that you are going to pull the Bite Block forward (toward you) using an isometric pull. You will only be using a small amount of resistance.

    **Note:** If you observe any evidence of jaw sliding or jutting, attempt to achieve the natural bite posture 3 times. If after 3 attempts the client continues to demonstrate jaw instability, return to Exercise B - Twin Bite Blocks for Jaw Stability.

3. While maintaining the natural bite posture, pull forward on the ends of the Bite Block using isometric resistance until you reach the goal of 15 seconds or the client fails to achieve the 15-second goal.

    **Note:** Failure is described as seen in any of the following scenarios:

    a. The client cannot maintain the hold on the Bite Block and it comes out of the mouth.

    b. The client uses any of the following compensatory postures to keep the Bite Block in his/her mouth: moves forward, turns the head, moves backward, uses whole body tension to maintain the bite on the therapy tool, or uses hands to hold the jaw closed.

4. Make a note of the 15-second success or the number of seconds achieved before failure.

5. Criteria for Success: Hold the natural bite posture on the #2 Bite Block for 15 seconds while maintaining the isometric pull, without any evidence of compensatory patterns, 1 time.

Step #2    One of the following scenarios will be evident:

1.  If the client can achieve the criteria for success, place a check mark in the chart below as indicated. You have now completed your jaw height level 2 assessment. Congratulations– but you are not done yet! To continue your assessment you will now use Bite Block #3 to repeat the three exercises:

**Exercise A - Bite Block**

**Exercise B - Twin Bite Blocks for Symmetrical Jaw Stability**

**Exercise C - Bite Block for Jaw Stability**

### TalkTools® Jaw Grading Bite Block Assessment and Treatment Form

| Tool | A. Bite Block Exercise | B. Twin Bite Block for Symmetrical Jaw Stability Exercise | C. Bite Block for Jaw Stability Exercise |
|---|---|---|---|
| Prerequsite Bite and Hold | __✓__ 10 sec. R __✓__ 10 sec L (1X) | | |
| Bite Block #2 | __✓__ 15 sec. R __✓__ 15 sec L (1X) | __✓__ 15 sec. R & L (1X) | __✓__ 15 sec. (1X) |
| Bite Block #3 | _____ 15 sec. R _____ 15 sec L (1X) | _____ 15 sec. R & L (1X) | _____ 15 sec. (1X) |

a.  If the client can achieve the criteria for success on all three exercises using the #3 Bite Block, repeat the sequence using the #4 Bite Block, then the #5 Bite Block, then the #6 Bite Block and finally the #7 Bite Block.

b.  Continue to fill in the TalkTools® Jaw Grading Bite Block Assessment and Treatment Form as described until your client fails on any of the sequential exercises. When failure occurs, enter that information on the form. Your assessment is now complete. Proceed to Using the Correct Diagnostic Term on page 99.

2.  If the client does not meet the 15-second criteria for success using the #2 Bite Block, enter the highest number of seconds achieved before failure in the chart on the next page as indicated in the following example. Your assessment is now complete. Proceed to Using the Correct Diagnostic Term on page 99.

# TalkTools® Jaw Grading Bite Block Assessment and Treatment Form

| Tool | A. Bite Block Exercise | B. Twin Bite Block for Symmetrical Jaw Stability Exercise | C. Bite Block for Jaw Stability Exercise |
|---|---|---|---|
| Prerequsite Bite and Hold | __✓__ 10 sec. R __✓__ 10 sec L (1X) | | |
| Bite Block #2 | __✓__ 15 sec. R __✓__ 15 sec L (1X) | __✓__ 15 sec. R & L (1X) | _10_ 15 sec. (1X) |

97

# HOW TO EVALUATE JAW STABILITY

These exercises are presented in chronological order. Follow the chart from left to right, beginning with Bite Block #2 and the exercise entitled **A. Bite Block Exercise.** If the client achieves the Criteria for Success, progress to **B. Twin Bite Block Exercise** using Bite Block #2. If the client achieves the Criteria for Success, progress to **C. Bite Block for Jaw Stability Exercise** using Bite Block #2. If the client achieves the Criteria for Success in this exercise, repeat the same sequence of exercises using Bite Blocks #3 through #7 as listed in the chart below. Exercise **D. Jaw Exerciser** will only be used if the client achieves the Criteria for Success for all exercises involving Bite Blocks #2 through #7.

**Note:**

As soon as the client fails to reach the Criteria for Success for any of the exercises listed below, you have completed your jaw diagnostic workup. Therapy will begin at this level.

## TalkTools® Jaw Grading Bite Block Assessment and Treatment Form

| Tool | A. Bite Block Exercise | | B. Twin Bite Block Exercise | C. Bite Block for Jaw Stability Exercise |
|---|---|---|---|---|
| **Bite Block #2** | _____ 15 sec. R | _____ 15 sec. L (1x) | _____ 15 sec. R & L (1x) | _____ 15 sec. (1x) |
| **Bite Block #3** | _____ 15 sec. R | _____ 15 sec. L (1x) | _____ 15 sec. R & L (1x) | _____ 15 sec. (1x) |
| **Bite Block #4** | _____ 15 sec. R | _____ 15 sec. L (1x) | _____ 15 sec. R & L (1x) | _____ 15 sec. (1x) |
| **Bite Block #5** | _____ 15 sec. R | _____ 15 sec. L (1x) | _____ 15 sec. R & L (1x) | _____ 15 sec. (1x) |
| **Bite Block #6** | _____ 15 sec. R | _____ 15 sec. L (1x) | _____ 15 sec. R & L (1x) | _____ 15 sec. (1x) |
| **Bite Block #7** | _____ 15 sec. R | _____ 15 sec. L (1x) | _____ 15 sec. R & L (1x) | _____ 15 sec. (1x) |

### D. Jaw Exerciser

Jaw Exerciser #1 _____ Position #1, 15 seconds (1x) _____ Position #2, 15 seconds (1x) _____ Position #3, 15 seconds (1x)

Jaw Exerciser #2 _____ Position #1, 15 seconds (1x) _____ Position #2, 15 seconds (1x) _____ Position #3, 15 seconds (1x)

**Criteria for Success:** Completes all of the above    **Diagnosis:** Symmetrical Jaw Stability    **Treatment:** No jaw exercises are needed

© Copyright 1993 Sara Rosenfeld-Johnson, M.S., CCC-SLP Speech-Language Pathologist Rev. 04/08

# Using the Correct Diagnostic Term

Now that you have completed your diagnosis and filled out the appropriate information on the TalkTools® Jaw Grading Bite Block Assessment and Treatment Form, it will be necessary to translate that information into a diagnostic term for report writing and to then decide on the most appropriate treatment plan. From the following diagnostic terms, choose the one that best describes your client's performance. Once you have chosen the appropriate diagnostic term proceed to **Treatment - Therapeutic Technique**, on page 102.

1. **Jaw Stability at Jaw Heights #2 through #7**: This client has met the criteria for success for all exercises at each jaw height level using TalkTools® Jaw Grading Bite Blocks #2 through #7.

   Example: Jaw stability at Jaw Heights #2 through #7

## TalkTools® Jaw Grading Bite Block Assessment and Treatment Form

| Tool | A. Bite Block Exercise | B. Twin Bite Block for Symmetrical Jaw Stability Exercise | C. Bite Block for Jaw Stability Exercise |
|------|------------------------|-----------------------------------------------------------|------------------------------------------|
| Prerequsite Bite and Hold | ✓ 10 sec. R ✓ 10 sec L (1X) | | |
| Bite Block #2 | ✓ 15 sec. R ✓ 15 sec L (1X) | ✓ 15 sec. R & L (1X) | ✓ 15 sec. (1X) |
| Bite Block #3 | ✓ sec. R ✓ 15 sec L (1X) | ✓ 15 sec. R & L (1X) | ✓ 15 sec. (1X) |
| Bite Block #4 | ✓ 15 sec. R ✓ 15 sec L (1X) | ✓ 15 sec. R & L (1X) | ✓ 15 sec. (1X) |
| Bite Block #5 | ✓ 15 sec. R ✓ 15 sec L (1X) | ✓ 15 sec. R & L (1X) | ✓ 15 sec. (1X) |
| Bite Block #6 | ✓ 15 sec. R ✓ 15 sec L (1X) | ✓ 15 sec. R & L (1X) | ✓ 15 sec. (1X) |
| Bite Block #7 | ✓ 15 sec. R ✓ 15 sec L (1X) | ✓ 15 sec. R & L (1X) | ✓ 15 sec. (1X) |

2. **Symmetrical Jaw Weakness:** This next client has failed at any of the jaw levels in Exercise A - Bite Block. The failure has been at the same number of seconds on both the right and left sides, so both sides of the jaw demonstrate equal weakness at that jaw height.

Example: Symmetrical Jaw Weakness

## TalkTools® Jaw Grading Bite Block Assessment and Treatment Form

| Tool | A. Bite Block Exercise | B. Twin Bite Block for Symmetrical Jaw Stability Exercise | C. Bite Block for Jaw Stability Exercise |
|---|---|---|---|
| Prerequsite Bite and Hold | ✓ 10 sec. R ✓ 10 sec L (1X) | | |
| Bite Block #2 | ✓ 15 sec. R ✓ 15 sec L (1X) | ✓ 15 sec. R & L (1X) | ✓ 15 sec. (1X) |
| Bite Block #3 | ✓ sec. R ✓ 15 sec L (1X) | ✓ 15 sec. R & L (1X) | ✓ 15 sec. (1X) |
| Bite Block #4 | 9 15 sec. R 9 15 sec L (1X) | 15 sec. R & L (1X) | 15 sec. (1X) |

3. **Asymmetrical Jaw Weakness:** This next client has failed at any of the jaw height levels in Exercise A - Bite Block, but the failure occurs at a different number of seconds on the right side than on the left. This means that both sides of the jaw demonstrate weakness at that jaw height, but one side is weaker than the other.

Example: Asymmetrical Jaw Weakness

## TalkTools® Jaw Grading Bite Block Assessment and Treatment Form

| Tool | A. Bite Block Exercise | B. Twin Bite Block for Symmetrical Jaw Stability Exercise | C. Bite Block for Jaw Stability Exercise |
|---|---|---|---|
| Prerequsite Bite and Hold | ✓ 10 sec. R ✓ 10 sec L (1X) | | |
| Bite Block #2 | ✓ 15 sec. R ✓ 15 sec L (1X) | ✓ 15 sec. R & L (1X) | ✓ 15 sec. (1X) |
| Bite Block #3 | ✓ sec. R ✓ 15 sec L (1X) | ✓ 15 sec. R & L (1X) | ✓ 15 sec. (1X) |
| Bite Block #4 | 9 15 sec. R 13 15 sec L (1X) | 15 sec. R & L (1X) | 15 sec. (1X) |

4. **Asymmetrical Jaw Weakness – One Sided:** This next client has failed at any of the jaw height levels in Exercise A - Bite Block. However, failure only occurs on one side of the jaw, while at the same jaw height the client has met the 15-second criteria for success on the other side of the mouth. This means only one side of the jaw is weak.

Example: Asymmetrical Jaw Weakness – one sided

## TalkTools® Jaw Grading Bite Block Assessment and Treatment Form

| Tool | A. Bite Block Exercise | B. Twin Bite Block for Symmetrical Jaw Stability Exercise | C. Bite Block for Jaw Stability Exercise |
|---|---|---|---|
| Prerequsite Bite and Hold | ✓ 10 sec. R ✓ 10 sec L (1X) | | |
| Bite Block #2 | ✓ 15 sec. R ✓ 15 sec L (1X) | ✓ 15 sec. R & L (1X) | ✓ 15 sec. (1X) |
| Bite Block #3 | ✓ sec. R ✓ 15 sec L (1X) | ✓ 15 sec. R & L (1X) | ✓ 15 sec. (1X) |
| Bite Block #4 | 9 15 sec. R ✓ 15 sec L (1X) | _____ 15 sec. R & L (1X) | _____ 15 sec. (1X) |

# TREATMENT – Therapeutic Technique

Now that you have completed your diagnosis, filled out the appropriate information on the TalkTools® Jaw Grading Bite Block Assessment and Treatment Form, and chosen the most appropriate diagnostic term, it will be necessary to translate that information into a treatment program. You will begin at the highest level before failure, as noted on the TalkTools® Jaw Grading Bite Block Assessment and Treatment Form. Use the following diagnostic terms to identify the number of repetitions to be performed daily and the appropriate ratio of practice repetitions to be used with each of your clients:

## Diagnosis #1: Jaw Stability at Jaw Heights #2 through #7:

When a client has achieved the criteria for success for all exercises at each jaw height using TalkTools® Jaw Grading Bite Blocks #2 through #7, that client does not need to work on static strength at any given jaw height. None of the following exercises will be necessary.

## Diagnosis #2: Symmetrical Jaw Weakness:

Step #1

1. Symmetrical Jaw Weakness: For clients with this diagnosis you will be practicing the following ratio of repetitions: 1 unit = 1 time to the right side for every 1 time to the left, 10 times per day. For example, if the client fails on Exercise A - Bite Block, using the #4 Bite Block, at 9 seconds on the right side and 9 seconds on the left as described in the chart below, you would begin your therapy program at Exercise A - Bite Block. One unit would consist of one 9-second isometric pull to the right side, followed by one 9-second isometric pull to the left, and this unit would be practiced 10 times per day. The 10 repetitions can be completed at the same time or in smaller segments spread throughout the day, as long as 10 repetitions are completed daily.

### TalkTools® Jaw Grading Bite Block Assessment and Treatment Form

| Tool | A. Bite Block Exercise | B. Twin Bite Block for Symmetrical Jaw Stability Exercise | C. Bite Block for Jaw Stability Exercise |
|---|---|---|---|
| Prerequsite Bite and Hold | ✓ 10 sec. R ✓ 10 sec L (1X) | | |
| Bite Block #2 | ✓ 15 sec. R ✓ 15 sec L (1X) | ✓ 15 sec. R & L (1X) | ✓ 15 sec. (1X) |
| Bite Block #3 | ✓ sec. R ✓ 15 sec L (1X) | ✓ 15 sec. R & L (1X) | ✓ 15 sec. (1X) |
| Bite Block #4 | 9 15 sec. R 9 15 sec L (1X) | 15 sec. R & L (1X) | 15 sec. (1X) |

102

2. Place the tip of the indicated Bite Block on the surface of the left lower back molars, extending from the front of the mouth as performed in the diagnostic assessment. Instruct the client to use the natural bite posture to bite down on the Bite Block.

   **Note:** In the above example you would be using the #4 Bite Block.

3. Explain to the client that you are going to pull the Bite Block forward (toward you) using an isometric pull.

   **Note:** In the above example you would be pulling for 9 seconds.

4. Remove the Bite Block and repeat on the right side of the mouth.

5. Practice the prescribed unit, consisting of 1 time to the right for every 1 time to the left 10 times per day as homework for a minimum of one week. Increase in 1-second increments as your client achieves skills until you reach 14 seconds per side, 10 times.

6. Increase the duration of the isometric pull to 15 seconds per side, 1 time.

7. Criteria for Success: Hold the natural bite posture on the targeted Bite Block for 15 seconds while maintaining the isometric pull on both the left and right sides of the mouth, without any evidence of compensatory posturing, 1 time. (Criteria for success for **Exercise A - Bite Block**.)

Step #2

1. Enter this information on the TalkTools® Jaw Grading Bite Block Assessment and Treatment Form, as illustrated below:

## TalkTools® Jaw Grading Bite Block Assessment and Treatment Form

| Tool | A. Bite Block Exercise | B. Twin Bite Block for Symmetrical Jaw Stability Exercise | C. Bite Block for Jaw Stability Exercise |
|---|---|---|---|
| Prerequsite Bite and Hold | _✓_ 10 sec. R _✓_ 10 sec L (1X) | | |
| Bite Block #2 | _✓_ 15 sec. R _✓_ 15 sec L (1X) | _✓_ 15 sec. R & L (1X) | _✓_ 15 sec. (1X) |
| Bite Block #3 | _✓_ sec. R _✓_ 15 sec L (1X) | _✓_ 15 sec. R & L (1X) | _✓_ 15 sec. (1X) |
| Bite Block #4 | _✓_ 15 sec. R _✓_ 15 sec L (1X) | ____ 15 sec. R & L (1X) | ____ 15 sec. (1X) |

2. If your client has been working with Bite Block #2, 3, 4, 5 or 6, you will now proceed to **Exercise B – Twin Bite Blocks for Symmetrical Jaw Stability** and follow the directions as described on page 93. Remember to follow the chronology of

exercises by working horizontally across the TalkTools® Jaw Grading Bite Block Assessment and Treatment Form, using each Bite Block level as you progress through the TalkTools® Jaw Grading Bite Block exercise program.

**Exercise A – Bite Block Exercise**

**Exercise B – Twin Bite Blocks for Symmetrical Jaw Stability**

**Exercise C – Bite Block for Jaw Stability**

**Diagnosis #3: Asymmetrical Jaw Weakness:**

Step #1

1. <u>Asymmetrical Jaw Weakness:</u> For clients with this diagnosis you will be practicing the following ratio of repetitions: 1 unit = 2 times to the weaker side for every 1 time to the stronger side, 10 times per day. For example, if the client fails on **Exercise A - Bite Block**, using the #3 Bite Block, at 3 seconds on the left side and 8 seconds on the right as shown in the chart below, you would begin your therapy program at **Exercise A - Bite Block**, where one unit would consist of one 3-second isometric pull to the left side followed by one 8-second isometric pull to the right, followed by one 3-second pull to the left, 10 times per day. The 10 repetitions can be completed at the same time, or in smaller segments spread throughout the day, as long as the 10 repetitions are completed daily.

### TalkTools® Jaw Grading Bite Block Assessment and Treatment Form

| Tool | A. Bite Block Exercise | B. Twin Bite Block for Symmetrical Jaw Stability Exercise | C. Bite Block for Jaw Stability Exercise |
|---|---|---|---|
| Prerequsite Bite and Hold | ✓ 10 sec. R ✓ 10 sec L (1X) | | |
| Bite Block #2 | ✓ 15 sec. R ✓ 15 sec L (1X) | ✓ 15 sec. R & L (1X) | ✓ 15 sec. (1X) |
| Bite Block #3 | *8* sec. R *3* 15 sec L (1X) | 15 sec. R & L (1X) | 15 sec. (1X) |

2. Place the tip of the indicated Bite Block on the surface of the left lower back molars, extending from the front of the mouth as performed in the diagnostic assessment. Instruct the client to use a natural bite posture to bite down on the Bite Block.
   **Note**: In the above example you would be using the # 3 Bite Block.

3. Explain to the client that you are going to pull the bite block forward (toward you) using an isometric pull.

**Note:** In the above example you would be pulling for 3 seconds on the left side.

4. Remove the Bite Block and repeat on the right side of the mouth.

   **Note:** In the above example you would be pulling for 8 seconds on the right side.

5. Remove the Bite Block and repeat on the left side of the mouth.

   **Note:** In the above example you would again be pulling for 3 seconds on the left side.

6. Practice the prescribed unit, consisting of 2 times to the weaker side for every 1 time to the stronger side, 10 times per day as homework for a minimum of one week. Increase in 1-second increments as your client achieves skills until you reach 14 seconds per side, 10 times.

7. Increase the duration of the isometric pull to 15 seconds per side, 1 time.

8. <u>Criteria for Success:</u> Hold the natural bite posture on the targeted Bite Block for 15 seconds while maintaining the isometric pull on both the left and right sides of the mouth, without any evidence of compensatory posturing, 1 time. (Criteria for success for **Exercise A - Bite Block**.)

<u>Step #2</u>

1. Enter this information on the TalkTools® Jaw Grading Bite Block Assessment and Treatment Form, as illustrated below:

### TalkTools® Jaw Grading Bite Block Assessment and Treatment Form

| Tool | A. Bite Block Exercise | B. Twin Bite Block for Symmetrical Jaw Stability Exercise | C. Bite Block for Jaw Stability Exercise |
|------|------------------------|------------------------------------------------------------|-------------------------------------------|
| Prerequsite Bite and Hold | ✓ 10 sec. R ✓ 10 sec L (1X) | | |
| Bite Block #2 | ✓ 15 sec. R ✓ 15 sec L (1X) | ✓ 15 sec. R & L (1X) | ✓ 15 sec. (1X) |
| Bite Block #3 | ✓ sec. R ✓ 15 sec L (1X) | _____ 15 sec. R & L (1X) | _____ 15 sec. (1X) |

2. If your client has been working with Bite Blocks #2, 3, 4, 5 or 6, you will now proceed to **Exercise B – Twin Bite Blocks for Symmetrical Jaw Stability** and follow the directions as described on page 93. Remember to follow the chronology of exercises by working horizontally across the TalkTools® Jaw Grading Bite Block Assessment and Treatment Form, using each Bite Block level as you progress through the TalkTools® Jaw Grading Bite Block exercise program.

**Exercise A – Bite Block Exercise**
**Exercise B – Twin Bite Blocks for Symmetrical Jaw Stability**
**Exercise C – Bite Block for Jaw Stability**

Step #1

1. Asymmetrical Jaw Weakness – One Sided: For clients with this diagnosis you will be practicing the following ratio of repetitions: 1 unit = 1 time to the weaker side only, 10 times per day. For example, if the client fails on **Exercise A - Bite Block** using the #6 Bite Block at 6 seconds on the left side, but meets the 15-second criteria for success on the right side as described in the chart below, you would begin your therapy program at **Exercise A - Bite Block** using a unit consisting of one 6-second isometric pull to the left side only, 10 times per day. The 10 repetitions can be completed at the same time or in smaller segments spread throughout the day, as long as the 10 repetitions are completed daily.

**TalkTools® Jaw Grading Bite Block Assessment and Treatment Form**

| Tool | A. Bite Block Exercise | B. Twin Bite Block for Symmetrical Jaw Stability Exercise | C. Bite Block for Jaw Stability Exercise |
|---|---|---|---|
| Prerequsite Bite and Hold | __✓__ 10 sec. R __✓__ 10 sec L (1X) | | |
| Bite Block #2 | __✓__ 15 sec. R __✓__ 15 sec L (1X) | __✓__ 15 sec. R & L (1X) | __✓__ 15 sec. (1X) |
| Bite Block #3 | __✓__ sec. R __6__ 15 sec L (1X) | _____ 15 sec. R & L (1X) | _____ 15 sec. (1X) |

2. Place the tip of the indicated Bite Block on the surface of the lower back molars on the weak side of the mouth, extending from the front of the mouth as performed in the diagnostic assessment. Instruct the client to use the natural bite posture to bite down on the Bite Block.
   **Note:** In the above example you would be using the #6 Bite Block.

3. Explain to the client that you are going to pull the Bite Block forward (toward you) using an isometric pull.
   **Note:** In the above example you would be pulling for 6 seconds on the left side, as this is the side determined to be "weak" during the assessment.

4. Practice the prescribed unit, consisting of 1 time to the weak side only, 10 times per day as homework for a minimum of one week. Increase in 1-second increments as your client achieves skills until you reach 14 seconds, 10 times.

5. Increase the duration of the isometric pull to 15 seconds per side, 1 time.

6. Criteria for Success: Hold the natural bite posture on the targeted Bite Block for 15 seconds while maintaining the isometric pull on both the left and right sides of the mouth, without any evidence of compensatory posturing, 1 time. (Criteria for success or **Exercise A - Bite Block**)

Step #2

1. Enter this information on the TalkTools® Jaw Grading Bite Block Assessment and Treatment Form, as illustrated below:

**TalkTools® Jaw Grading Bite Block Assessment and Treatment Form**

| Tool | A. Bite Block Exercise | B. Twin Bite Block for Symmetrical Jaw Stability Exercise | C. Bite Block for Jaw Stability Exercise |
|---|---|---|---|
| Prerequsite Bite and Hold | ✓ 10 sec. R ✓ 10 sec L (1X) | | |
| Bite Block #2 | ✓ 15 sec. R ✓ 15 sec L (1X) | ✓ 15 sec. R & L (1X) | ✓ 15 sec. (1X) |
| Bite Block #3 | ✓ sec. R ✓ 15 sec L (1X) | 15 sec. R & L (1X) | 15 sec. (1X) |

2. If your client has been working with Bite Blocks #2, 3, 4, 5 or 6, you will now proceed to **Exercise B – Twin Bite Blocks for Symmetrical Jaw Stability** and follow the directions as described on page 93. Remember to follow the chronology of exercises by working horizontally across the TalkTools® Jaw Grading Bite Block Assessment and Treatment Form, using each Bite Block level as you progress through the TalkTools® Jaw Grading Bite Block exercise program.

**Exercise A – Bite Block Exercise**

**Exercise B – Twin Bite Blocks for Symmetrical Jaw Stability**

**Exercise C – Bite Block for Jaw Stability**

# GUM CHEWING

Gum chewing, as an activity, is one of the most comprehensive techniques I have ever used. It addresses jaw, lip and tongue functioning. The only two criteria necessary to initiate a gum chewing program are the presence of at least two back molars (one on each side) and the ability to swallow without aspiration. Gum chewing can even be used with severely cognitively-impaired clients who cannot follow verbal directions but demonstrate an oral movement cause and effect understanding. In addition, clients who demonstrate any of the following habits will benefit from a gum chewing program: teeth grinding, thumb sucking, pacifier sucking, bottle sucking, tongue sucking, excessive mouthing of objects or clothing, biting and drooling.

Gum chewing can also be used to teach tongue retraction and tongue lateralization. When you instruct the client to chew with the lips closed, you will also be working on lip closure.

Clients who have sensory processing or sensory-based behavior disorders benefit from "gum chewing," as it helps to stabilize the body and to organize the sensory system.

The specific oral placement or movement goals are listed after each Step.

Suggestions

1. Before introducing this activity, speak with the parents to explain the importance of introducing gum chewing as it relates specifically to their child. Show them the entire hierarchy and explain that their child will be taught how to chew gum slowly and safely, without the danger of swallowing the piece of gum.

2. You will need to make a decision about what kind of gum you are going to use to implement this activity. Choose sugarless or sugared bubble gum. The texture will vary according to the type of gum you choose.

   a. Sugared gum starts out firmer and gets "gooey" over time. It requires more intensity and is used for shorter duration chewing.

   b. Sugarless gum starts out softer and gets firmer over time. It is used for clients who need to chew for longer periods of time.

   **Note:** The ultimate decision may depend on the client's dental health or dietary requirements.

3. Do not use gum chewing with clients who have diagnosed **TMJ** problems.

4. Gum chewing is used to improve jaw stability and to improve jaw grading.

   a. If the client has symmetrical instability in the jaw, chew the gum on alternating sides of the mouth when following the hierarchy.

108

- b. If the client is weak on both sides but is weaker on one side, chew two times to the weaker side for every one time to the stronger side.
- c. If the client has normal skills on one side and weakness on one side, chew only on the weak side.

5. Gum Chewing can be used to help organize the body and to improve attention to task.
6. WORK SLOWLY! If you try to progress too rapidly, the client may not succeed.
7. There are three components to every Step. Each segment should be given equal importance:
    - a. <u>Introduction:</u> Introducing the gum to the client
    - b. <u>Task:</u> Gum in the mouth
    - c. <u>Disposal:</u> Placing the gum in the garbage or trash can
8. Each Step is repeated daily until the task is mastered.
9. Steps #1 through #7 are done sitting down facing the client.
10. <u>Homework:</u> Establish during the session where the client fails on the hierarchy. Practice that Step at the highest level of successful repetitions for at least one week before moving on to the next level or Step.

## Step #1

1. <u>Introduction:</u> Have the client help unwrap the bubble gum.
2. <u>Task:</u>
    - a. Break off 1/2 of the piece and form into a 1" roll as pictured below. You may wrap this roll in a piece of gauze or organza if you are nervous about the client biting off a piece of the gum and swallowing it.

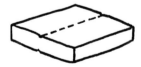  

    - b. Place the end of the 1" roll on the surface of the back molar(s) on the client's left side; do not release the roll of gum at any time during this Step.
    - c. Instruct the client to bite down on the piece of gum. Use assisted jaw stability to establish a **natural bite** if necessary.
    - d. Instruct the client: "Open your mouth" and "Give it back to me." With less cognitively intact clients, you may have to assist the client in opening his/her

mouth as you remove the gum.  Use a paper towel or cotton towel to remove the saliva from the gum roll.

    e.  Repeat the same procedure on the right side of the mouth on the surface of the lower back molar(s).

    f.  Continue to dry off and reshape the gum as you alternate from left side placement to right side placement.

    g.  Work until the client tires, becomes bored or does not cooperate.

3.  <u>Disposal:</u>  Put the gum in the paper towel and go to the garbage can with the client.  Have the client drop the gum into the garbage can independently; assist only if necessary.  Make sure to verbally praise the client for throwing the gum in the garbage can when he/she is finished chewing it.

<u>Goal:</u>  Eliminate the association of chewing the gum then swallowing the gum

## Step #2

1.  <u>Introduction:</u>  Have the client remove the gum from the wrapper and dispose of the wrapper in the garbage can.

2.  <u>Task:</u>

    a.  Break off 1/2 of the piece and form into a 1" roll.  You may continue to wrap this roll in gauze or organza if you are nervous about the client biting off a piece of the gum and swallowing it.

    b.  Place the end of the gum roll on the surface of the lower back molar (s) on the left side.  Instruct the client to bite two times and release the gum.  Use the verbal cues, "Bite, open, bite, open, now give it back," as you remove the gum.

    c.  Repeat the procedure on the surface of the lower molar(s) on the right side.

    d.  Increase the number of bites followed by a "give it back," up to 10 per side.

    e.  Continue to dry off and reshape the gum roll after each side is completed.

    f.  Do not release the gum roll at any time.

    g.  Continue until the client becomes bored or uncooperative.

3.  <u>Disposal:</u>  Have the client put the used gum in the paper towel and put it in the garbage can.

<u>Goals:</u>

    1.  Eliminate the association of chewing the gum then swallowing the gum

2. Improve symmetrical jaw mobility

3. Improve jaw stability and grading

4. Improve placement for tongue retraction

5. Eliminate negative oral habits

6. Decrease drooling

Step #3

1. Introduction: Have the client remove the bubble gum from the wrapper and deposit the wrapper in the garbage can.

2. Task:

   a. Break off 1/2 of the piece of bubble gum and form it into a ball.

   b. Tell the client you will be putting the gum in his/her mouth, and it is to be chewed and then given back.

   c. Put the gum in the client's mouth on the surface of either lower back molar(s). Press down slightly to secure the gum and then remove your finger. Use the verbal cues, "Chew, chew, chew - give the gum back to me," to pattern the client's movements. Remove the gum from the client's mouth.

   **Note:** When the client intentionally releases the gum when you say, "Give it back," congratulate yourself.

   d. Reshape the gum and repeat on the other side of the mouth.

   e. Continue to alternate from one side to the other side (1 unit), 10 times.

3. Disposal: Have the client put the used gum in the paper towel and put it in the garbage can.

   Goals:

      1. Eliminate the association of chewing the gum then swallowing the gum

      2. Improve symmetrical jaw mobility

      3. Improve jaw stability and grading

      4. Improve placement for tongue retraction

      5. Eliminate negative oral habits

      6. Decrease drooling

Step #4:

Confirm that the client is able to lateralize food across midline before attempting this

Step. If the client cannot lateralize across midline, remain at Step #3 until you teach tongue lateralization across midline through your feeding intervention.

1. Introduction: Have the client remove the bubble gum from the wrapper and deposit the wrapper in the garbage can.

2. Task:

   a. Use 1/2 of the piece of bubble gum formed into a ball.

   b. Have the client put the gum into the mouth on either back molar(s) and chew it on that side 5 times.

   c. Instruct the client to move it to the other side and "give it back to me." The client does not need to be able to count; you can tap out 5 times.

   d. Reshape the gum and repeat the task on the other side of the mouth.

   e. Repeat 10 times on each side of the mouth.

3. Disposal: Have the client put the used gum in the paper towel and put it in the garbage can.

   Goals:

   1. Eliminate the association of chewing the gum then swallowing the gum

   2. Improve symmetrical jaw mobility

   3. Improve jaw stability and grading

   4. Improve placement for tongue retraction

   5. Eliminate negative oral habits

   6. Decrease drooling


Step #5

1. Introduction: Use the same procedure described above.

2. Task:

   a. Use 1/2 of the piece of bubble gum formed into a ball.

   b. Have the client put the ball into the mouth and chew it on the back molar(s) on either side 5 times, move it to the other side and chew it 5 more times. You may have to assist in reshaping.

   c. Alternate 5 chews on each side until the gum becomes very soft. Instruct the client: "Give it back to me."

   d. Add the other half of the original piece of gum by wrapping the soft piece around the new piece to increase the texture.

   e. Continue until the gum can be chewed in this manner for 2 minutes.

3. <u>Disposal:</u>  Use the same procedure as described above.

   <u>Goals:</u>

   1. Improve symmetrical jaw mobility
   2. Improve jaw stability and grading
   3. Improve placement for tongue retraction
   4. Eliminate negative oral habits
   5. Decrease drooling
   6. Improve tongue lateralization skills

## Step #6

1. <u>Introduction:</u>  Use the same procedure as described above.

2. <u>Task:</u>

   a. Instruct the client to bite off a piece of the bubble gum, chew it until it gets soft, then bite off a new piece until the entire piece is in the mouth.

   b. Intermittently remind the client to move the gum to the other side.

3. <u>Disposal:</u>  After three minutes, instruct the client to take the gum out of the mouth, put it in the paper towel, take it to the garbage can and throw it away.

   <u>Goals:</u>

   1. Improve symmetrical jaw mobility
   2. Improve jaw stability and grading
   3. Improve placement for tongue retraction
   4. Eliminate negative oral habits
   5. Decrease drooling
   6. Improve tongue lateralization skills

## Step #7

1. <u>Introduction:</u>  Use the same procedure as described above.

2. <u>Task:</u> Allow the client to move freely around the room to practice Step #6 for one minute.

3. <u>Disposal:</u>  Use the same procedure as described above.

## Step #8

1. <u>Introduction:</u> Use the same procedure as described above.

2. <u>Task:</u>

113

a. Allow the client to move freely around the room to practice Step #6 for two minutes.

b. Increase the number of minutes while closely monitoring to ensure that the client does not become so distracted as to swallow the gum.

3. Disposal: Use the same procedure as described above.

Step #9

1. Introduction: Use the same procedure as described above.

2. Task:

a. Start with one piece of bubble gum chewed with the lips closed for 5 minutes.

b. Increase by 1 minute each day until you reach 15 minutes.

c. This activity can be paired with television watching or with a fine motor task.

3. Disposal: By this time, the client should be able to decide when and how to dispose of the gum.

Goals:

1. Improve symmetrical jaw mobility

2. Improve jaw stability and grading

3. Improve placement for tongue retraction

4. Eliminate negative oral habits

5. Decrease drooling

6. Improve tongue lateralization skills

7. Improve placement for lip closure

# SECTION 2 - LIP ACTIVITIES

There is a difference between an inability to close the lips secondary to weak or unstable lip musculature verses the same inability secondary to weak or unstable jaw musculature. It will be important for you to determine if one or both of these causative factors is present. If jaw musculature is weak, you will use a combination program of jaw activities and lip activities. If the jaw musculature is strong enough to support grading, you will be able to concentrate on lip activities alone. Prior to any work on lip closure, it will be critical to determine if the client is able to breathe adequately through the nose. If the client is an **obligatory mouth breather**, a referral to a medical professional will be necessary to determine if the condition is permanent or can be corrected with medical or surgical intervention.

The reduction or elimination of drooling is a goal for many of our clients. It is important to understand the components of an inability to control saliva prior to working on its elimination. There are four possible issues that can result in drooling. Any one of them, or any combination of the four, will result in the client's inability to control saliva buildup. Let's try a little experiment. We will pretend we have low muscle tone.

1.  Sit in a straight back chair, with your legs slightly apart. Push your pelvis back as you scoot your bottom forward on the chair.
2.  Lean forward with your arms resting weakly on your legs.
3.  Open your mouth to breathe as you look down at your legs.
4.  Remain in that position for one minute. What happened? If you followed each of these directions, you who are cognitively intact, with at least adequate muscle control, are now drooling.

## Here are the four contributing factors:

1.  Hypotonicity - body and head posture
2.  Open mouth posture, secondary to mouth breathing, reduced muscle strength or muscle skill levels
3.  Hyposensitivity/responsivity - Inability, or reduced ability, to feel the saliva
4.  Inability or difficulty retracting saliva back over the tongue to initiate a swallow
    As you can see, working on lip closure is only one part of a comprehensive saliva control program. The other issues will have to be addressed simultaneously for successful reduction or elimination of drooling.

The activities in this chapter follow the hierarchy of lip development as outlined in Chapter 2. Please refer to that hierarchy before introducing any of the following lip activities.

115

# CRUMBS

Since awareness is a prerequisite for volitional movement, awareness of lip placement is a critical component of reducing drooling, improving feeding and improving speech clarity. This activity will address the awareness component of lip closure in the same way that "Bubble Blowing," Step #1, addresses lip awareness.

The specific oral placement or movement goals are listed after each Step.

Suggestions:

1.  Prior to this activity, determine food preferences and identify any food allergies or dietary restrictions.

2.  You will need a non-latex glove and crumbs of varying textures to implement this activity.

3.  Begin with crumbs that are light in weight and are finely ground, such as graham crackers. As skill levels increase, add weight by using coarser textures. Adding weight increases awareness.

4.  Use a glove which is tight fitting to avoid a negative reaction from your client. If your hand is not sweating within a minute of putting the glove on, it is probably not tight enough. Conversely, you do not want to cut off your circulation. Choose gloves that fit you, not One Size Fits All.
    **Note:**
    a.  Remember to wash the powder off the gloves after you put them on your hands.
    b.  Flavored gloves may be used as long as the "taste" does not interfere negatively with the existing sensory system.
    c.  Vinyl or other non-latex gloves must be used for clients with latex intolerance.

5.  In contrast to many of the activities in this book, there is no suggested number of repetitions or Criteria for Success. The technique has been established to increase awareness and should be used prior to lip activities which require volitional control.

6.  This technique has been very successful with clients who:
    a.  Have difficulty effecting jaw elevation for lip closure
    b.  Are fixing in a low jaw posture
    c.  Are drooling secondary to a flaccid open mouth posture

Step #1

1. Place the crumbs in the palm of your gloved hand.
2. Use a non-flavored chapstick or Carmex as an adhesive. If your client is drooling, you will not have to worry about an adhesive. It is already there for you.
3. Firmly press the crumbs onto the client's mouth, as pictured below.

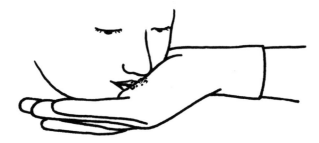

4. Remove your hand and wait for any attempt at closure. Wipe the crumbs off your client's mouth immediately with a soft cloth, working gently towards midline, and repeat this Step.
5. Repeat this technique until the closure response is no longer present, the client tires of the technique, the client's tongue protrudes to retrieve the crumbs, or ideally until the client closes the lips in anticipation of the "feel" of the crumbs.

**Note:** A tactile cue can be used with clients who immediately protrude the tongue: use **assisted jaw elevation** prior to putting the crumbs on the lips.

Goals:
1. Improve awareness on the lips as a prerequisite for lip closure placement
2. Work on elevating the jaw from an open mouth posture

Target Phonemes:     / m, b, p /

Step #2

1. Increase the texture of the crumbs. Adding weight will not only increase awareness but will require increased effort to effect lip closure.
2. Make sure to talk about how the client's lips feel. Through this awareness technique, volitional movements can eventually be elicited through verbal directions.
3. Immediately follow this activity with the appropriate lip activity to address your goal of either lip closure or lip rounding (Horn Blowing, Straw Drinking, Tongue Depressor, etc.).

Goals:

1. Improve awareness on the lips as a prerequisite for volitional lip closure placement
2. Work on elevating the jaw from an open mouth posture
3. Associate the "feel" of lip closure with the verbal direction, "Close your lips."

   Target Phonemes:  / m, b, p /

# SINGLE-SIP CUP DRINKING

In addition to including feeding goals in your Program Plan, clients can be using "Single-Sip Cup Drinking" in the oral placement/movement activity component of the Plan. For clients with no identifiable feeding difficulties, this technique can assist in the development of volitional lip closure through repetition and the development of muscle memory.

The specific oral placement or movement goals are listed after each Step.

Suggestions:

1. To implement this activity you will need a cup with a straight edge to create a firmer lip seal on the cup rim.
2. Prior to introducing this activity, take a food/drink preference inventory.
   a. If the client has difficulty swallowing certain textures, that information should be paramount in determining which liquid you choose for the single-sip technique.
   b. Applesauce, yogurt and fruit purees can be thinned to make them "liquids" for clients who do not have swallowing difficulties but prefer those tastes to other liquids.
   c. Soda and similar sugared drinks, although not a parent's first choice, may be a motivating factor for a resistive client or clients with the diagnosis of hyposensitivity/responsivity.
3. Homework:  Establish during the session where the client fails on the hierarchy. Practice that Step at the highest level of successful repetitions for at least one week before moving onto the next level or Step.

Step #1

1. Fill a cup with six ounces of the **favorite liquid**.
   **Note:**  For pre-independent clients, I use a "cut-out" cup or one I make from a plastic container (e.g., shampoo container, soft plastic cup, etc.). The amount of liquid will depend on the cup capacity (up to six ounces).
2. Depending on age and skill levels, determine if the client must be assisted with drinking or can be allowed to perform this technique independently.
3. Use a quick wrist action to introduce the liquid into the client's mouth. Wait for lip closure, or assist with lip closure, as required by the client's needs.
4. Wait for a swallow, then reintroduce the cup immediately.

5. Repeat this rapid-feed technique until all of the liquid has been consumed.

6. <u>Criteria for Success:</u> Continue one time per day until lip closure is no longer considered a therapeutic goal.

   **Note:** This will complete the "Single-Sip Cup Drinking" technique, unless you have a further goal of:

   a  Creating a "standard swallow"

   b  Establishing a retracted tongue-tip elevation posture with lip closure as an habitual posture at rest

<u>Goals:</u>

1. Improve awareness on the lips as a prerequisite for volitional lip closure placement

2. Work on elevating the jaw from an open mouth posture

3. Improve lip closure placement and muscle memory

<u>Target Phonemes:</u>        / m, b, p /

<u>Step #2</u>

1. Fill a straight rimmed cup with eight ounces of a favorite liquid.  By this Step, the client will probably be self-feeding.  If not, you will have to continue holding the cup.

2. Instruct the client:

   a. "Take a single-sip."

   b. "Remove the cup as you close your lips."

   c. "Elevate your tongue-tip to the alveolar ridge."

   d. "Freeze."

   e. "Swallow without moving your tongue tip or opening your lips."

3. After the first swallow instruct the client to open his/her mouth to make sure that the tongue tip is still on the alveolar ridge.

4. Repeat these instructions until all eight ounces have been consumed correctly.

5. <u>Criteria for Success:</u> Continue one time per day for one month.

   <u>Goals:</u>

1. Improve lip closure placement and muscle memory

2. Increase tightening of the mentalis muscle system

3. Associate verbal directions with physical movements

4. Improve placement for tongue-tip elevation skills

5. Improve jaw stability and grading

6. Introduce a standard swallow pattern

<u>Target Phonemes:</u>  / m, b, p, f, v, r / and all phonemes which require tongue retraction

## <u>Step #3</u>

1. Fill a straight-mouthed cup with 16 ounces of a favorite liquid.

2. Repeat the technique described in Step #2 with all 16 ounces at one sitting.

3. <u>Criteria for Success:</u>  Continue one time per day for three months.

    <u>Goals:</u>

    1. Improve lip closure placement and muscle memory

    2. Increase tightening in the mentalis muscle system

    3. Associate verbal directions with physical movements

    4. Improve placement for tongue-tip elevation skills

    5. Improve jaw stability and grading

    6. Introduce a standard swallow pattern

    <u>Target Phonemes:</u>  / m, b, p, f, v, r / and all phonemes which require tongue retraction

# KISSES

Kissing is an activity that can be used to reduce hypersensitivity/responsivity or tactile defensiveness on the face and lips. Kissing is also beneficial for increasing awareness on the face and lips for clients who are hyposensitive/responsive, especially for those clients who have drooling problems, secondary to an inability to feel saliva buildup on the lips, or who maintain the mouth in a chronic open mouth posture.

The specific oral placement or movement goals are listed after each Step.

Suggestions:

1.  Prior to introduction of this activity, determine your target lip placement for the kiss. If your goal is to reduce or to increase sensitivity, the placement may not be important. If, however, your goal is to improve lip closure or rounding, the appropriate lip placement will have to be maintained throughout the activity.

2.  Since you will be working on more than one technique during a session, and if your goal includes a specific lip placement (closure or rounding), using a horn blowing activity prior to "Kissing," may improve placement performance.

3.  You will need non-latex gloves, a stuffed animal or doll, a puppet, five finger puppets, a permanent marker, a water-based marker, yarn, and a pair of scissors to implement this activity.

4.  The kissing activity will be explained as it would be used to address sensitivity issues. As you become more familiar with this technique, you will find you do not have to use each Step when your goals relate solely to lip placement.

5.  This activity has been used successfully with clients who are initially resistant to the use of gloves during therapy. As you know, gloves are a must when we plan to touch a client who is drooling, or when we enter a client's mouth for feeding, oral placement/movement therapy or to establish placement for phoneme production.

    **Note:** Refer to the activity entitled, "Crumbs," for a discussion of glove size and type.

6.  Homework: Establish during the session where the client fails on the hierarchy. Practice that Step at the highest level of successful repetitions for at least one week before moving onto the next level or Step.

Step #1

1.  Prior to introducing this technique, ask the parents or caregiver to bring a few of the

client's favorite stuffed animals or dolls to this session.  You will return them at the end of each session.   At the same time, ask the parents or caregiver if they have any puppets at home.  If not, ask them to purchase at least one puppet and to let the client play with these toys at home.  Your goal is to have items the child will readily touch.

2. Begin by allowing the client to hold and play with the stuffed animals or dolls. Observe how much touch can be tolerated and specifically how much is allowed on the face and lips.

3. Introduce yourself into the play by touching the stuffed animal/doll as the child continues to play.

   **Note:** It is important to go very slowly at this point.  You are trying to establish trust; if you move too quickly, you may ruin a very effective technique.

4. If the client shows any level of discomfort as a result of your introduction, pull back and try again in a few minutes.

   **Note:** Sometimes it is helpful if you have your own stuffed animal/doll which you can use for parallel play to reduce the client's discomfort level.

   Goal: Establish acceptance of these stuffed animals/dolls as therapy tools

## Step #2

1. Continue to use the stuffed animals/dolls the child brings from home.

2. Using the same "approach-pull back" technique described in Step #1, work slowly until the client allows you to not only touch the stuffed animal/doll while he/she is playing with it, but allows you to hold it independently and then return it to the client.

   Goal: Establish acceptance of these stuffed animals/dolls as therapy tools

## Step #3

1. Continue to use the stuffed animals/dolls the child brings from home.

2. Using the "approach-pull back" technique, work until the client allows you to hold the stuffed animal/doll and use it to "kiss" the client.  With highly defensive clients, work from kissing their arms and legs first. Work slowly to the shoulders, back of head, neck and finally onto the face using firm touch.  Make the kissing sound as you pretend the stuffed animal/doll is kissing the client.

3. When you are able to use the stuffed animal/doll to kiss the client's lips, you can progress to Step #4.

Goals:

1. Establish acceptance of the stuffed animal/doll as a therapy tool
2. Increase placement for lip closure or lip rounding

**Note:** If your goal is to work on lip closure or on lip rounding and not on acceptance of touch, encourage the client to kiss the stuffed animal/doll back. Homework would be to kiss one or a number of stuffed animals/dolls, 50 times per day, to master the motor plan for lip closure or lip rounding placement.

Step #4

1. Ask the parent to send in a puppet instead of a stuffed animal/doll.
2. Place the puppet on your hand and work towards kissing the client with the puppet's mouth. Continue to make the kissing sound.
3. Pretend your hand is getting cold or the inside of the puppet is uncomfortable to you. Explain your problem to the client. Solve the problem by putting on a tight non-latex glove in front of the client. Put the puppet back on your hand and immediately return to the "kissing" activity.

   **Note:** It is important to use a tight glove as the surplus on the tips of your fingers is frequently the reason clients do not like gloves.

   Goals:

   1. Establish acceptance of the puppet as a therapy tool
   2. Establish acceptance of the glove under the puppet
   3. Increase tolerance to touch
   4. Decrease oral hypersensitivity/responsivity
   5. Decrease tactile defensive behaviors

Step #5

1. Once the client willingly accepts the kiss from the puppet, progress to finger puppets.
2. Place one finger puppet on each of your five gloved fingers. Have each finger puppet kiss the client's lips. Make sure the client sees you are wearing a glove.

   Goals:

   1. Establish acceptance of the glove under the finger puppet
   2. Increase tolerance to touch
   3. Decrease oral hypersensitivity/responsivity
   4. Decrease tactile defensive behaviors

124

Step #6

1. Once the client willingly accepts the kiss from the finger puppets, progress to glove puppets.

2. Before the client enters the room, make the glove puppet:

   a. Put on a tight non-latex glove.

   b. Use permanent marker to draw eyes, nose and mouth on each finger.

   c. Glue yarn hair onto each finger tip.

3. Repeat the "kissing" activity using these glove puppets.

4. Once the client willingly accepts the kiss from the glove puppets, begin to give each puppet a haircut. Progress very slowly. After each trim, have that puppet kiss the client's lips.

5. Work until the puppets are bald.

   Goals:

   1. Tolerate the use of gloves on the client's lips

   2. Decrease oral hypersensitivity/responsivity

   3. Decrease tactile defensive behaviors

Step #7

1. Use water-based markers to draw eyes, nose and mouth on each bald glove puppet.

2. Go to the sink, with the client to "give the puppets a bath."

3. After each bald glove puppet is bathed, kiss the client's lips with that gloved finger.

4. Complete this technique by using your clean gloved pointer finger to kiss the client's teeth.

   Goals:

   1. Tolerate the use of gloves on and within the oral cavity

   2. Decrease oral hypersensitivity/responsivity

   3. Decrease tactile defensive behaviors

125

# HUMMING #2

Most children love music.  By associating humming with listening to music or marching to music, you are capitalizing on that love of music.  Humming increases awareness on the lips and encourages prolongation of lip closure (i.e., placement/muscle memory), both components of saliva control.  This activity also establishes a controlled nasal airflow, a prerequisite for the activity entitled, "Oral-Nasal Contrasts."

The specific oral placement or movement goals are listed after each Step.

Suggestions:

1.  Whenever possible, it is the goal of intervention to teach nasal breathing.  When a client is breathing through the nose, the jaw can then be elevated to assist in lip closure.  The tongue is then retracted within the oral cavity.  Humming can be used to establish a closed mouth resting posture.

2.  You will need a music source and a mirror to implement this technique.

3.  Homework: Establish during the session where the client fails on the hierarchy. Practice that Step at the highest level of successful repetitions for a least one week before moving on to the next level or Step.

Step #1

1.  Use a familiar audio tape or CD for this activity.

2.  Instruct the client to hum as long as he/she hears the tape.  "Hum" along with the client.  Monitor to ensure the client is not using compensatory body fixing (i.e., shoulder elevation, etc.) to produce the airflow.  If the client cannot produce the humming without these compensatory patterns, return to the abdominal muscle activities (i.e., "Horn Blowing", "Bubble Blowing," etc.)

3.  Begin with two-second segments.  Turn off the music between segments.  Between segments the lips are allowed to open.

4.  Use a mirror and verbal cues to remind the client to keep the lips closed.

5.  Criteria for Success: Have the client complete 10 two-second humming tasks in rapid succession without a break.

     Goals:

       1.  Increase awareness of the lips

       2.  Teach placement for lip closure

       3.  Teach nasal airflow control

       4.  Reduce drooling

126

Target Phonemes:

    a.  Lip closure:  / m, b, p /

    b.  Nasal resonance: / m, n, ŋ (ng) /

## Step #2

1. Increase the duration of the humming in each breath group.

2. Criteria for Success:  Work until the client can hum an entire children's song, without opening the lips.

Goals:

1. Increase awareness on the lips

2. Teach placement for lip closure

3. Teach nasal airflow control

4. Reduce drooling

Target Phonemes:

    a.  Lip closure:  / m, b, p /

    b.  Nasal resonance: / m, n, ŋ (ng) /

# SPONGE-BALSA-TONGUE DEPRESSOR

Many clients are unable to achieve lip closure placement through verbal and/or visual cueing, secondary to improper jaw height. For clients who have a diagnosis of Cerebral Palsy, Moebius syndrome or Traumatic Brain Injury, it is very difficult or even impossible to achieve volitional jaw and lip closure. In addition to working on jaw closure activities with Bite Blocks, this technique will assist in achieving lip closure placement.

The specific oral placement or movement goals are listed after each Step.

Suggestions:

1. You will need three items to implement this activity: a make-up sponge, a piece of lightweight balsa wood and a flavored or non-flavored tongue depressor.
2. The make-up sponges used in this activity are light, thick and absorbent. Cut a round 1/2" wide make-up sponge into five equal pieces. The three center pieces will be in a rectangle shape approximately 1 1/2" by 1/2", as pictured below.

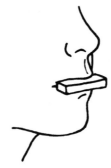

**Note:** For clients with severe drooling problems, the sponge will adhere to the lips and expand with the saliva. They should be washed thoroughly or discarded after each practice session.

3. Balsa is a lightweight wood used in making model airplanes. It can be found in a variety of shapes and thicknesses. Find a piece that is thinner, yet heavier, than the make-up sponge.
4. Use a flavored tongue depressor. For clients who drool, the flavor of the tongue depressor will combine with the saliva, thereby, increasing awareness of the saliva. You will notice that these clients will begin to "soup in" the flavored saliva during this activity.
5. This activity can only be done when the jaw is in a relaxed posture. Massage and vibration can be used to inhibit compensatory jaw "fixing" postures.
6. Homework: Establish during this session where the client fails on the hierarchy. Practice that Step at the highest level of successful repetitions for a least one week before moving on to the next level or Step.

Step #1

1. Use massage or vibration to relax the jaw. Once "fixing" is eliminated, use assisted jaw stability to establish a 3 to 4 level jaw height.
   **Note:** Do not attempt this activity when "fixing" is present.
2. Place the rectangular piece of make-up sponge between the lips, extending out the sides of the mouth to increase awareness. Talk about how the sponge feels between the lips. Release your hold on the sponge.

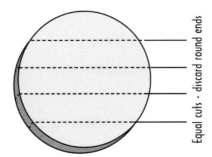

3. Criteria for Success: The client will maintain lip closure on the make-up sponge for 25 seconds, 3 times.
   Note: Monitor to ensure the client is not holding his/her head back to rely on gravity.
   Goals:
   1. Improve awareness of the lips
   2. Teach placement for volitional lip closure
   3. Reduce drooling
   4. Teach jaw-lip dissociation

   Target Phonemes: / m, b, p / and the vocalic / r /

Step #2

1. Transition to the pre-cut piece of balsa wood - 2" x 1/2" x 1/2."
2. Place the balsa wood between the lips horizontally, extending out the sides of the mouth, in the same position as pictured above. Use assisted jaw stability initially to establish the desired jaw height.
3. Eliminate the superimposed jaw stability while the client continues to hold the piece of balsa wood between the closed lips.
4. Work in a slight chin tuck to inhibit gravity from assisting in this activity.
5. Criteria for Success: The client will hold the piece of balsa wood between the closed lips for 25 seconds, 3 times, before progressing on to Step #3.
   **Note:** Monitor to ensure that the client is not holding his/her head back to rely on gravity.

Goals:

1. Improve awareness of the lips

2. Teach placement for volitional lip closure

3. Reduce drooling

4. Teach jaw-lip dissociation

Target Phonemes: / m, b, p / and the vocalic / r /


Step #3

1. Transition to the flavored tongue depressor.

2. Place the flat side of the tongue depressor between the closed lips, extending from the sides of the mouth.

3. Use assisted jaw stability initially to establish a 2 to 3 level jaw height. Eliminate the assisted stability after the tongue depressor has been placed between the closed lips.

**Note:** If the client is clenching his/her teeth initially, the posture is acceptable. However, in order to achieve the criteria for success, you will have to eliminate the teeth clenching. The teeth should be touching lightly together or in close proximity.

4. Criteria for Success: Instruct the client to hold the tongue depressor between the closed lips (without teeth clinching) for 25 seconds, 3 times.

**Note:** Progress from this activity to the technique entitled, "Tongue Depressor for Lip Closure."

Goals:

1. Improve awareness of the lips

2. Teach placement for volitional lip closure

3. Reduce drooling

4. Teach jaw-lip dissociation

Target Phonemes: / m, b, p / and the vocalic / r /

# TONGUE DEPRESSOR FOR LIP CLOSURE

Production Criteria for / m , b , p /

This activity is designed to improve awareness, placement, strength/stability, and muscle memory for the lip closure needed to teach the bilabial phonemes / m, b, p /. In addition, clients who demonstrate a w/r substitution may be using the orbicularis-oris muscles instead of the mentalis muscle system. This technique will improve mentalis muscle placement, strength/stability and muscle memory for standard production of /r/ and the vocalic /r/. Since prolonged lip closure is a component of saliva control, this activity should be used with clients who are drooling.

The specific oral placement or movement goals are listed after each Step.

Suggestions:

1. You may begin this activity at Step #1 with clients who can hold a tongue depressor between the closed lips, extending from the sides of the mouth, without teeth clenching, for one second.

2. For clients who do not possess sufficient lip closure/strength to hold the tongue depressor for one second, return to the activity entitled: "Sponge-Balsa-Tongue Depressor."

3. For clients who can only hold the tongue depressor between the closed lips with teeth clenching, thereby, using compensatory jaw assistance, begin with Step #1 of this activity. If compensatory teeth clenching cannot be eliminated by the conclusion of Step #1, return to the jaw stability activity prior to introducing the remainder of this activity.

4. You will need flavored or non-flavored tongue depressors, a package of pennies and some tape to implement this activity.

5. Prerequisite: "Jaw Grading Bite Block Exercises." Complete the Criteria for Success for Bite Block #2 and Bite Block #3.

6. Homework: Establish during the session where the client fails on the hierarchy. Practice that Step at the highest level of successful repetition for at least one week before moving on to the next level or Step.

Step #1

1. Place the single flavored tongue depressor horizontally between the closed lips, extending from the sides of the mouth, as pictured:

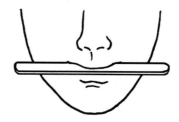

2. <u>Criteria for Success:</u> Instruct the client to hold the tongue depressor for 25 seconds, 3 times.

**Note:**
   a. If this posture can only be taught with teeth together placement, accept that compensatory posture initially. Elimination of compensatory teeth clenching must be achieved before progressing to Step #2.
   b. Monitor to ensure the client is using jaw-lip dissociation. The jaw should be stable, and no sliding or jutting forward should be seen. The lips should remain flat and relaxed. They should not be tightened in a compensatory "fixing" pattern.

<u>Goals:</u>
   1. Increase awareness of the lips
   2. Improve placement for lip closure
   3. Reduce drooling
   4. Improve mobility in the mentalis muscle system for placement of the /r/ and vocalic / r /

<u>Target Phonemes:</u> / m, b, p, r / and vocalic / r /


<u>Step #2</u>
   1. Place a single penny on the top surface at each end of the tongue depressor. Secure each penny with a piece of tape.
   2. Place the tongue depressor with the two attached pennies horizontally between the closed lips, extending from the sides of the mouth, as pictured below:

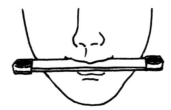

   3. <u>Criteria for Success:</u> Instruct the client to hold the tongue depressor, with a slight chin tuck, for 25 seconds, 3 times, before progressing to Step #3.

Goals:

1. Increase awareness of the lips

2. Improve placement for lip closure

3. Reduce drooling

4. Improve mobility in the mentalis muscle system for placement of the /r/ and vocalic / r /

Target Phonemes:  / m, b, p, r / and vocalic / r /

## Step #3

1. Introduce the standard production of / m /, / b /, / p / in isolation.

   **Note:** Prior to this step, complete auditory awareness and discrimination for your target phoneme.

2. Instruct the client to put his/her lips together, as practiced with the tongue depressor, and to say either / m, b, or p /.

3. Criteria for Success:  Repeat the standard production of your target phoneme 50 times, without using the tongue depressor for placement, before progressing to the word level.

   **Note:** When working with an apraxic client, keep the tongue depressor in the client's mouth during phoneme production to assist in motor planning for the / m, b, or p /.

4. Choose any traditional therapy approach you feel comfortable with to work on carryover.

   Goals:

   1. Increase awareness of the lips

   2. Improve placement for lip closure

   3. Reduce drooling

   4. Improve mobility in the mentalis muscle system for placement of the /r/ and vocalic / r /

   Target Phonemes:  / m, b, p, r / and vocalic / r /

## Step #4

1. Place another penny on top of each of the existing pennies, for a total of  4 pennies. Secure with tape.

2. Place this "mini-barbell" between the lips as described in Step #2.

133

3.  Instruct the client to hold this position for 25 seconds, 3 times.

4.  <u>Criteria for Success:</u> Increase the number of pennies, one per side, holding for 25 seconds, 3 times, until you have a total of 16 pennies on the "mini-barbell."

    **Note:** When the client can hold the 16 pennies for 25 seconds, 3 times, you have developed significant strength/muscle memory in the mentalis muscle system for standard lip placement for /r/ and vocalic / r /.

    <u>Goals:</u>

    1.  Increase awareness of the lips
    2.  Improve lip closure
    3.  Reduce drooling
    4.  Improve mobility in the mentalis muscle system for placement of the /r/ and vocalic / r /

    <u>Target Phonemes:</u>  / m, b, p, r / and vocalic / r /

# FINE MOTOR TASKS WITH LIP CLOSURE

Many of our clients have the necessary skill levels to achieve lip closure during a therapy session or when they are reminded to close their lips. Sometimes clients with fine motor deficits in the mouth exhibit fine motor deficits in the hands. For these clients, achieving lip closure can be very difficult while concentrating on fine motor hand tasks. Associating a lip closure activity with a fine motor hand task during the therapy session can help to transition this skill into a habit. In addition to addressing lip closure, this technique has been used to teach retraction of saliva for drooling control.

The specific oral placement or movement goals are listed after each Step.

Suggestions:

1. If the client is receiving occupational therapy, speak to that therapist. Find out the highest level fine motor task the client can perform successfully. Use this identified task as the fine motor component of this activity.

2. You will need either flavored or non-flavored tongue depressors to implement this activity.

3. Using a flavored tongue depressor will flavor the saliva. Adding taste to the saliva will increase awareness. This awareness will trigger volitional retraction of the saliva to stimulate a swallow.

4. Since this technique helps to control drooling, transitioning it into the classroom has been less difficult than expected. The reduced drooling enables the client to hand in papers that are neater, thereby engaging the teacher's cooperation in implementing the use of the activity. Another benefit to using this technique in the classroom is that reduced drooling often triggers improved social acceptance with peers.

5. Homework: Establish during the session where the client fails on the hierarchy. Practice that Step at the highest level of successful repetitions for at least one week before moving on to the next level or Step.

Step #1

1. With the client seated in a stable posture, present the fine motor task on a flat table surface or on an inclined board which will encourage a slight chin tuck.

2. Place a flavored tongue depressor horizontally between the client's closed lips, as described in the activity entitled, "Tongue Depressor for Lip Closure."

135

3. Instruct the client to keep both lips closed on the tongue depressor as the fine motor task is completed (i.e., put a peg in a peg board). Between trials, the tongue depressor can be removed from between the lips.

4. Talk about how it "feels" to keep the lips closed on the tongue depressor while he/she is working.

5. Criteria for Success: Repeat this task 10 times before progressing to Step #2.

   Goals:

   1. Associate lip closure with fine motor task completion
   2. Reduce drooling
   3. Encourage nose breathing
   4. Teach habitual closed mouth posture at rest
   5. Stimulate awareness of sensory input

   Target Phonemes: / m, b, p , r / and the vocalic / r /


Step #2

1. Transition the use of the tongue depressor between the closed lips to fine motor task completion outside of the therapy room, both at home and in the client's classroom.

2. Criteria for Success: Increase the length of time the client maintains the tongue depressor between the closed lips by one second per trial to ensure success up to one minute.

   Goals:

   1. Associate lip closure with fine motor task completion
   2. Reduce drooling
   3. Encourage nose breathing
   4. Teach habitual closed mouth posture at rest

   Target Phonemes: / m, b, p, r / and the vocalic / r /


Step #3

1. Increase the number of seconds, as awareness and skill levels improve, up to five minutes.

2. Criteria for Success: Remove the tongue depressor and work on holding the lips together during a fine motor task. Begin with one minute and work up to 15 minutes.

   **Note:** Initially, you may have to use visual or verbal cues to help in the transition.

Goals:
1. Associate lip closure with fine motor task completion
2. Reduce drooling
3. Encourage nose breathing
4. Teach habitual closed mouth posture at rest

Target Phonemes: / m, b, p, r / and the vocalic / r /

# STRAW HIERARCHIES

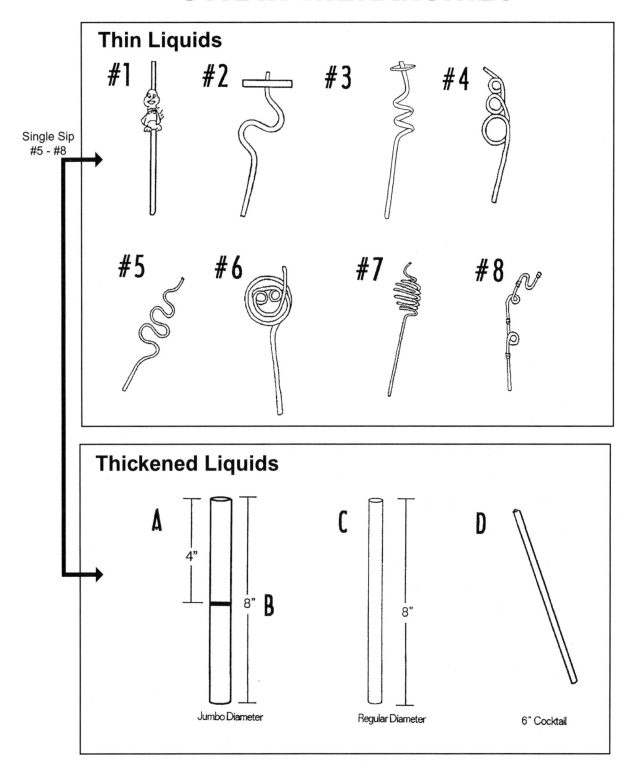

137

# STRAW DRINKING HIERARCHY

Therapeutic straw drinking should be incorporated into the Program Plan when any of your therapy goals include tongue or lip mobility, placement, position or strength. This technique can be used with very young children, as well as with adults. It has been used successfully with clients who evidence severe cognitive deficits and for those with normal intelligence. **Therapeutic straw drinking** is the best technique I have found to achieve tongue stability and dissociation. It addresses the **eight levels of tongue grading**.

The specific oral placement or movement goals are listed after each Step.

Suggestions:

1. You will need the TalkToolsTherapy ® Straw Kit to implement this activity.

2. The Straw Hierarchy for Thin Liquids is designed as a home program. Each new straw or Step should be introduced by the therapist and should then be sent home for daily practice.

3. The straws can be used in a juice box, with a TalkToolsTherapy ® Recessed Lid Drinking Cup, or in any other stable container. When using the very complex straws, with cognitively impaired or very young clients, you may want to use a sports bottle. Place part or all of the straw inside the container. This positioning will make the drinking posture more stable and will reduce the likelihood of spillage.

4. When drinking through the targeted straw on the hierarchy becomes "easy," the criteria for introducing the next straw on the hierarchy, has been met.

5. Ideally, the client will drink all thin liquids, all of the time, through the targeted straw on the hierarchy.

6. When this program is introduced to children under two to three years of age or those with significant placement and movement disorders, it may take longer to complete all of the straws in the hierarchy.

7. A video entitled *Straws as Therapy Tools* by Sara Rosenfeld-Johnson, SLP, teaches the technique and the reasons for its inclusion in a therapy program. It is designed for therapists, parents, teachers, etc., to ensure each step is introduced and practiced correctly.

8. Homework: Establish during the session where the client fails on the hierarchy. Practice that Step at the highest level of successful repetitions for at least one week before moving onto the next level or Step. It is important that the client has his/her own set of straws to ensure the appropriate level is being practiced daily.

# STRAW HIERARCHY FOR THIN LIQUIDS

Step #1

1. Begin with Straw #1.

   **Note:** As you become more familiar with this technique, you may choose to enter the Straw Drinking Hierarchy at a higher level, based upon the client's skill levels.

2. Use only thin liquids: Water, juice, milk, etc. (You will never use thickened liquids with these straws.)

   **Note:**

   a. Prior to using any food-based therapy technique, determine if there are any swallowing deficits, food allergies or other dietary limitations.

   b. Very slightly thickened liquid may be used only if swallowing difficulties have been identified.

3. Allow the client to drink any thin liquid through a regular straw independently for 2 to 3 seconds.

4. Place your thumb and pointer finger next to the client's lips where the straw enters the mouth, as pictured below.

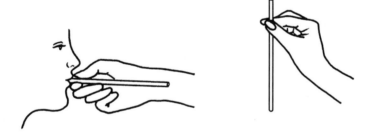

5. Remove the straw and measure the amount of straw that was in the client's mouth.

   **Note:** This measurement will allow you to determine if the client is biting on the straw or using a suckling pattern to draw the liquid through the straw. Your goal is to inhibit this suckle in favor of a lip protrusion with tongue retraction drawing posture.

6. Use the length identified in #4 of this Step to measure from the **lip block** on Straw #1 to the tip of the straw. Cut off the remaining portion of the straw tip. File the cut end with a nail file to make it smooth.

   **Note:** If the client has placed the entire tip of the straw up to the lip block in his/her mouth, you will not have to cut the straw at this time.

7. Criteria for Success: Send this straw home for one week. The client should be encouraged to drink all thin liquids through this straw. Either **single sips** or **repetitive draws** are acceptable.

    Goal: Establish acceptance of Straw #1 as a therapy tool

## Step #2

1. Use the same #1 straw the client used for homework.
2. Cut the straw tip by 1/4". Do not let the client observe this procedure.

    **Note:** When you use this technique with severely impaired clients, you may be cutting the straw in only 1/8" segments and remaining on that level for many weeks.

3. Instruct the client to drink a small juice box or three ounces of another appropriate liquid to establish he/she can perform straw drinking of liquids in this new manner.
4. Criteria for Success: Send this straw home for a minimum of one week. Either single sips or repetitive draws are acceptable.

    Goals:

    1. Improve placement for lip rounding
    2. Improve placement for tongue retraction
    3. Improve jaw stability and mobility
    4. Work toward independent self-feeding

    Target Phonemes:

    a. Lip rounding placement for:  / w,  o, u, ʊ, ɔ, ʃ(sh), ʧ(ch),  ʤ(j) /
    b. Tongue retraction placement for:  / m, b, p, f, v, k, g, t, d, n, s, z, l, r /

## Step #3

1. Continue to cut the tip of the straw in 1/4" increments until the entire tip is only 1/4" long.

    **Note:** The tongue may still be slightly protruded with some clients at the 1/4" level.

2. After each new cut, allow at least one week for the client to practice at each skill level.
3. Criteria for Success: Continue until drinking through the #1 straw cut to 1/4" above the lip block is easy for the client. Either single sips or repetitive draws are acceptable.

Goals:

1. Improve placement for lip rounding
2. Improve placement for tongue retraction
3. Improve jaw stability and mobility
4. Work toward independent self-feeding

Target Phonemes:

a. Lip rounding: / w, o, u, ʊ, ɔ, ʃ(sh), tʃ(ch), ʤ(j) /
b. Tongue retraction: / m, b, p, f, v, k, g, t, d, n, s, z, l, r /

## Step #4

1. Use Straw #2. Secure the lip block 1/4" from the tip of the straw. Place a rubber band under the lip block to secure its position if necessary.
   **Note:** This straw will never be cut.
2. Instruct the client to drink at least three ounces of any thin liquid before sending the new straw home for practice. Monitor to ensure the client is using lip protrusion with tongue retraction to draw the liquid up the length of the straw.
3. Criteria of Success: Do not progress to Step #5 until the client is drinking all thin liquids easily through Straw #2. Carryover to snacks and to all meals should be established before progressing to the next Step. Either single sips or repetitive draws are acceptable.
   Goals:
   1. Improve placement for lip rounding
   2. Improve placement for tongue retraction
   3. Improve jaw stability and mobility
   4. Work toward independent self-feeding

Target Phonemes:

a. Lip rounding: / w, o, u, ʊ, ɔ, ʃ(sh), tʃ(ch), ʤ(j) /
b. Tongue retraction: / m, b, p, f, v, k, g, t, d, n, s, z, l, r /

## Step #5

1. Introduce and use Straw #3 in the same manner as described above. Remember to present this new straw with the lip block only 1/4" from the straw tip.
2. Criteria for Success: Progress to Step #6 after the client can drink all thin liquids easily through Straw #3 at meals and snacks. Either single sips or repetitive draws are acceptable.

Goals:

1. Improve placement for lip rounding
2. Improve placement for tongue retraction
3. Improve jaw stability and mobility
4. Work towards independent self-feeding

Target Phonemes:

a. Lip rounding: / w, o, u, ʊ, ɔ, ʃ(sh), ʧ(ch), ʤ(j) /
b. Tongue retraction: / m, b, p, f, v, k, g, t, d, n, s, z, l, r /

Step #6

1. Introduce and use Straw #4 in the same manner as described above. Remember to present this new straw with the lip block (first twist) only 1/4" from the straw tip. In this case you will have to pre-cut the straw to 1/4" above the first twist.

2. Criteria for Success: Progress to Step #7 after the client can drink all thin liquids easily through Straw #4 at meals and snacks. Either single sips or repetitive draws are acceptable.

Goals:

1. Improve placement for lip rounding
2. Improve placement for tongue retraction
3. Improve jaw stability and mobility
4. Work toward independent self-feeding

Target Phonemes:

a. Lip rounding: / w, o, u, ʊ, ɔ, ʃ(sh), ʧ(ch), ʤ(j) /
b. Tongue retraction: / m, b, p, f, v, k, g, t, d, n, s, z, l, r /

Step #7

1. By this point, the client should be drinking with a lip protrusion/tongue retraction draw. There should be no evidence of inter-dental tongue protrusion during straw drinking. If any tongue protrusion is evident, return to a lower level on the Straw Hierarchy to teach that goal.

2. Introduce Straw #5 by allowing the client to drink a three ounce juice box independently. Observe to ensure the appropriate lip protrusion/tongue retraction is being used habitually.

**Note:** This straw does not have a lip block; one should not be added.

**Note:** If you are working with a client who will require help to achieve the appropriate position and/or to maintain the appropriate position, secondary to gross motor or fine motor limitations, continue supplying support throughout the remainder of this activity. Consultation with a physical therapist or an occupational therapist should be considered if you are unsure how to progress.

3.  After you have established the client is using the appropriate drawing technique, transition to a "single-sip technique."  Change the instructions as follows:
    a.  Place the straw between your lips.
    b.  Draw in the liquid until you feel it in your mouth.
    c.  Remove the straw but do not swallow the liquid.
    d.  Close your lips as you put your tongue tip up, just behind your front top teeth.
    e.  Freeze.
    f.  Now swallow the liquid without moving your tongue-tip.
    g.  Open your mouth, your tongue-tip should still be up behind your top teeth.

**Note:** For our clients with cognitive impairment, use the following instructions:
    a.  Place the straw between your lips.
    b.  Draw in the liquid until you feel it in your mouth.
    c.  Remove the straw.
    d.  Close your lips.
    e.  Swallow.

4.  Send Straw #5 home for practice only when the complete technique described above in #3 of this Step has been taught (single draw and swallow technique).

5.  Criteria for Success: Progress to Step #8 when the client can drink all thin liquids easily through Straw #5, as described above, using the single draw and swallow technique, at all meals and snacks.

Goals:
    1.  Improve placement for lip rounding and protrusion
    2.  Improve placement for tongue retraction
    3.  Improve jaw stability as a prerequisite for jaw-lip-tongue dissociation
    4.  Introduce a standard swallow pattern which inhibits tongue protrusion
    5.  Work toward independent self-feeding

Target Phonemes:
    a.  Lip rounding: / w,  o, u, ʊ, ɔ, ʃ(sh), ʧ(ch),  ʤ(j) /
    b.  Tongue retraction:  / m, b, p, f, v, k, g, t, d, n, s, z, l, r /

143

Step #8

1. Introduce and use Straw #6 in the same manner as described in Step #7.
   **Note:** This straw does not have a lip block; one should not be added.

2. Criteria for Success: Progress to Step #9, when the client can drink all thin liquids easily through Straw #6, as described above, using the single draw and swallow technique at all meals and snacks.

   Goals:
   1. Improve placement for lip rounding and protrusion
   2. Improve placement for tongue retraction
   3. Improve jaw stability as a prerequisite for jaw-lip-tongue dissociation
   4. Habituate a standard swallow pattern which inhibits tongue protrusion
   5. Work toward independent self-feeding

   Target Phonemes:
   a. Lip rounding: / w, o, u, ʊ, ɔ, ʃ(sh), ʧ(ch), ʤ(j) /
   b. Tongue retraction: / m, b, p, f, v, k, g, t, d, n, s, z, l, r /

Step #9

1. Introduce and use Straw #7 in the same manner as described in Step #7.
   **Note:** This straw does not have a lip block; one should not be added.

2. Criteria for Success: Progress to Step #10, when the client can drink all thin liquids easily through Straw #7, as described above, using the single draw and swallow technique, at all meals and snacks.

   Goals:
   1. Improve placement for lip rounding and protrusion
   2. Improve placement for tongue retraction
   3. Improve jaw stability as a prerequisite for jaw-lip-tongue dissociation
   4. Habituate a standard swallow pattern which inhibits tongue protrusion
   5. Work toward independent self-feeding

   Target Phonemes:
   a. Lip rounding: / w, o, u, ʊ, ɔ, ʃ(sh), ʧ(ch), ʤ(j) /
   b. Tongue retraction: / m, b, p, f, v, k, g, t, d, n, s, z, l, r /

Step # 10

1. Introduce and use Straw #8 in the same manner as described in Step #7.

**Note:** This straw does not have a lip block; one should not be added.

2. Criteria for Success: When the client is able to drink all thin liquids easily through Straw #8 at all meals and all snacks, tongue retraction should be sufficient to support tongue-back stability (i.e., back of tongue side spread) on the palate. Back of tongue side spread placement is needed for standard co-articulation and speech clarity.

Goals:

1. Improve placement for lip rounding and protrusion
2. Improve placement for back of tongue side spread
3. Improve jaw stability as a prerequisite for jaw-lip-tongue dissociation
4. Habituate a standard swallow pattern which inhibits tongue protrusion
5. Work toward independent self-feeding

Target Phonemes:

a. Lip rounding: / w, o, u, ʊ, ɔ, ʃ(sh), tʃ(ch), ʤ(j) /
b. Tongue retraction: / m, b, p, f, v, k, g, t, d, n, s, z, l, r /


## STRAW HIERARCHY FOR THICKENED LIQUIDS

(Introduce at the same time as Straw #5 on the Straw Drinking Hierarchy for Thin Liquids.)


Step #1

1. Begin with Straw A for Thickened Liquids (i.e., jumbo straw). Cut the jumbo straw to 4". A lip block should not be necessary, if you have worked through Straw #4 on the Straw Drinking Hierarchy for Thin Liquids.

   **Note:** This technique is introduced at the same time as straw #5 on the Straw Hierarchy for Thin Liquids is introduced, not before. These straws are used only one time per day for drinking three to four ounces of the targeted thickened liquid.

2. Use three ounces of nectar or a liquid of the same consistency as nectar.

   **Note:** Prior to using any food-based therapy technique, determine if there are any swallowing deficits, food allergies or other dietary limitations.

3. Place the container of nectar on the table in front of the client.

4. Instruct the client to lean forward and down to drink the nectar through the straw. The client can use either a single draw/swallow or repetitive draw/swallow. Working in this posture will increase tongue resistance, thereby increasing tongue retraction and lingual grading.

   **Note:** If the client cannot perform this task utilizing lip protrusion and tongue retraction to effect the draw, return to the Straw Drinking Hierarchy for Thin Liquids.

145

5. Make a list of similarly textured liquids the client can use for practice until your next session.

   **Note:** Thin liquids can be thickened slightly with SimplyThick™, infant cereals or agar, or purees can be thinned with water or juice.

6. Criteria for Success: Drink three to four ounces of the nectar one time per day through Straw A on the Straw Drinking Hierarchy for Thickened Liquids, which has been cut to 4" in length, for a minimum of one week or until it is easy, before progressing to Step #2.

   Goals:

   1. Improve placement for lip protrusion
   2. Improve placement for tongue retraction and grading
   3. Improve jaw-lip-tongue dissociation
   4. Work toward independent self-feeding

   Target Phonemes:

   a. Lip rounding: / w, o, u, ʊ, ɔ, ʃ(sh), ʧ(ch), ʤ(j) /
   b. Tongue retraction within the oral cavity: / m, b, p, f, v, k, g, t, d, n, s, z, l, r /

## Step #2

1. Continue to use Straw A for thickened liquids, cut to the 4" length.
2. Increase the texture of the food source to a puree consistency.
3. Criteria for Success: Drink three to four ounces of puree consistency one time per day through Straw A on the Straw Drinking Hierarchy for Thickened Liquids, which has been cut to 4" in length, for a minimum of one week or until it becomes easy, before progressing to Step #3.

   Goals:

   1. Improve placement for lip protrusion
   2. Improve placement for tongue retraction and grading
   3. Improve jaw-lip-tongue dissociation
   4. Work toward independent self-feeding

   Target Phonemes:

   a. Lip rounding: / w, o, u, ʊ, ɔ, ʃ(sh), ʧ(ch), ʤ(j) /
   b. Tongue retraction within the oral cavity: / m, b, p, f, v, k, g, t, d, n, s, z, l, r /

## Step #3

1. Continue to use Straw A, cut to the 4" length, for thickened liquids.
2. Increase the texture of the food source to a yogurt consistency.

**Note:** Avoid yogurts with fruit pieces, as they will clog the straw or may be aspirated. Be sure to be aware of the client's food likes and dislikes and of the existence of any allergies.

3. Criteria for Success: When the client is able to drink three to four ounces of this texture easily one time per day, for a minimum of one week, progress to Step #4.

   Goals:
   1. Improve placement for lip protrusion
   2. Improve placement for tongue retraction and grading
   3. Improve jaw-lip-tongue dissociation
   4. Work toward independent self-feeding

   Target Phonemes:
   a. Lip rounding: / w, o, u, ʊ, ɔ, ʃ(sh), ʧ(ch), ʤ(j) /
   b. Tongue retraction within the oral cavity: / m, b, p, f, v, k, g, t, d, n, s, z, l, r /

## Step #4

1. Continue to use Straw A, cut to the 4" length, for thickened liquids.
2. Increase the texture of the food source to a pudding consistency.
3. Criteria for Success: When the client is able to drink six ounces of this texture easily one time per day, for a minimum of one week, progress to Step #5.

   Goals:
   1. Improve placement for lip protrusion
   2. Improve placement for tongue retraction and grading
   3. Improve jaw-lip-tongue dissociation
   4. Work toward independent self-feeding

   Target Phonemes:
   a. Lip rounding: / w, o, u, ʊ, ɔ, ʃ(sh), ʧ(ch), ʤ(j) /
   b. Tongue retraction within the oral cavity: / m, b, p, f, v, k, g, t, d, n, s, z, l, r /

## Step #5

1. From this point on you will only be changing the straw, not the consistency of the thickened liquid. In other words, for the remainder of this activity you will only use pudding or thickened liquids of pudding consistency.

2. Your goal for this Step will be to increase the length of the jumbo straw to its original 8" length (Straw B).

3. Place the container on the table in front of the client. Instruct the client to lean forward and down to drink the pudding consistency.

4. Criteria for Success: Drink three to four ounces of the pudding consistency through the 8" Straw B (jumbo straw) one time per day, for a minimum of one week or until it becomes easy, before progressing to Step #6.

Goals:

1. Improve placement for lip protrusion
2. Improve placement for tongue retraction and grading
3. Improve jaw-lip-tongue dissociation
4. Work toward independent self-feeding

Target Phonemes:

a. Lip rounding: / w, o, u, ʊ, ɔ, ʃ(sh), ʧ(ch), ʤ(j) /
b. Tongue retraction within the oral cavity: / m, b, p, f, v, k, g, t, d, n, s, z, l, r /

## Step #6

1. Introduce Straw C for thickened liquids. This is a regular diameter straw. It does not have a lip block. By this time in the hierarchy, the client should not need one to maintain a proper placement.

2. Use only pudding or pudding consistency textures for this Step.

3. Criteria for Success: When the client is able to drink three to four ounces of this texture easily one time per day, for a minimum of one week, progress to Step #7.

Goals:

1. Improve placement for lip protrusion
2. Improve placement for tongue retraction and grading
3. Improve jaw-lip-tongue dissociation
4. Work toward independent self-feeding

Target Phonemes:

a. Lip rounding: / w, o, u, ʊ, ɔ, ʃ(sh), ʧ(ch), ʤ(j) /
b. Tongue retraction within the oral cavity: / m, b, p, f, v, k, g, t, d, n, s, z, l, r /

148

## Step #7

1. Introduce Straw D for thickened liquids (6" cocktail straw).

2. This is a difficult Step, but it can be done with conscientious effort and motivation.

3. Wrap a rubber band ¼" to ½" from the straw tip to ensure the client does not put more than the top of the straw in the mouth.

4. Use only pudding or pudding consistency textures for this Step.

5. Instruct the client to drink the pudding as follows:

    a. "Place the straw between your lips."

    b. "Draw in the pudding until you feel it in your mouth."

    c. "Remove the straw but do not swallow the pudding."

    d. "Close your lips as you put your tongue-tip up, just behind your front top teeth."

    e. "Freeze."

    f. "Now swallow the puree without moving your tongue tip."

    g. "Open your mouth, your tongue-tip should still be up behind your top teeth."

6. When the client is able to drink three to four ounces of a pudding texture easily through this straw using the standard swallow posture, you have completed the activity.

Goals:

1. Improve placement for tongue retraction and lingual grading needed for the standard production of sibilants

2. Teach back of tongue side spread for the standard production of / r / and the variants of / r /

3. Improve jaw-lip-tongue dissociation

Target Phonemes: / s, z, ʃ(sh), tʃ(ch), ʤ(j), r /

# OO-EE (OO-EE-AH)

"OO-EE" is an activity that works on teaching jaw-lip dissociation. It is also used to teach transition of movement from lip protrusion to lip retraction for clients with motor planning problems (e.g., apraxia). Use the "OO-EE-AH" configuration for clients who are speaking in a "high jaw fixed" posture to increase relaxed mobility in the jaw.

The specific oral placement or movement goals are listed after each Step.

Suggestions:

1. Prior to introducing this activity, determine if the client has sufficient jaw stability to maintain the jaw in a stable posture while the lips move into protrusion or retraction. Initially, you may have to stabilize the jaw to assist in teaching the dissociated movement. If, despite repetitive attempts, the jaw continues to move in direct association with lip movements, return to jaw activities.

2. After the introduction of this activity, ask the client if he/she is experiencing any pain in the temporomandibular joint area. If so, do not use this technique.

3. Prerequisite: "Jaw Grading Bite Block Exercises." Complete the Criteria for Success for Bite Block #2 through Bite Block #5.

4. Homework: Establish during the session where the client fails on the hierarchy. Practice that Step at the highest level of successful repetitions for at least one week before moving onto the next level or Step.

Step #1

1. Instruct the client to say "OO" or to put his/her lips in the "OO" position. With some clients, you may want to use a round-mouthed horn to teach the "OO" position.

2. Criteria for Success: Have the client repeat the "OO" sound 10 times in succession without a break.

**Note:** Monitor to ensure the jaw is not jutting. If the only way the client can say "OO" is to jut the jaw or to clench the teeth together, return to jaw stability activities.

Goals:

1. Teach placement for lip rounding
2. Develop jaw-lip dissociation

Target Phonemes: Lip rounding: / w, o, u, ʊ, ɔ, ʃ(sh), tʃ(ch), ʤ(j) /

Step #2

1. Instruct the client to say "EE" or to put his/her lips in the "EE" position. You may have to give minimal assisted jaw support initially to inhibit any widening of the jaw, as pictured below.

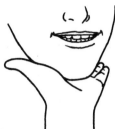

2. Criteria for Success: Have the client repeat the "EE" sound 10 times in succession without a break. Eliminate the jaw support and repeat the "EE" 10 times.
**Note:** Monitor to ensure the jaw is not jutting or sliding.
Goals:
   1. Teach placement for lip retraction
   2. Develop jaw-lip dissociation
Target Phonemes: Lip retraction vowels: / I (ih), i (ee), / and vocalic / r /

Step #3

1. Instruct the client to say "OO-EE" as one unit.
2. Criteria for Success: Have the client repeat the "OO-EE" unit 10 times without a break.
**Note:** The jaw should not slide or jut.
Goals:
   1. Teach placement for lip protrusion ⟶ lip retraction as a transition movement.
   2. Improve jaw-lip dissociation
   3. Facilitate motor planning
Target Phonemes:
   a. Lip rounding: / w, o, u, ʊ, ɔ, ʃ(sh), ʧ(ch), ʤ(j) /
   b. Lip retraction vowels: / I (ih), i (ee) / and vocalic / r /

Step #4

1. Instruct the client to say "OO-EE-AH" as one unit.
2. Criteria for Success: Have the client say the "OO-EE-AH" unit 10 times without a break.

Goals:

1. Inhibit "high jaw fixing" during connected speech utterances
2. Teach jaw-lip dissociation

# BUTTON PULL

This activity will address one of the components of insufficient saliva control: insufficient bilabial closure/reduced lip mobility. In addition, many clients who evidence interdental tongue protrusion during this function have reduced lip mobility. For example, the client may suckle on a straw rather than use lip protrusion with tongue retraction to draw up the liquid. Others may use the teeth or scrape purees from a spoon rather than removing the puree with the lips. As a result, the lips rest in an open mouth posture. This activity will address those clients and will also develop placement and mobility of the orbicularis-oris muscles as a prerequisite for standard speech sound production of: / w, o, u, ʊ, ɔ, ʃ(sh), tʃ(ch), dʒ(j) /

The specific oral placement or movement goals are listed after each Step.

Suggestions:

1. You will need five buttons of graduated sizes and dental floss to implement this activity.
2. Before introducing this technique, have five flat buttons of increasing size (3/8"; 1/2" [4/8"]; 5/8"; 3/4" [6/8"]; and 7/8") available, with a minimum of two holes in each. Place an 18" piece of dental floss in one of the holes and then through the other hole. When the lengths are even, tie a snug knot directly behind the button. You should now have two nine-inch lengths with the button in the middle. Repeat this procedure for each button. You should now have five buttons attached to five separate pieces of dental floss for this activity.
3. Remember to always hold on to the dental floss during this activity to ensure the button does not enter the oral cavity.
4. Homework: Establish during the session where the client fails on the hierarchy. Practice that Step at the highest level of successful repetitions for at least one week before moving onto the next level or Step.

Step #1

1. Instruct the client to close his/her teeth. Establish a natural bite. Measure the distance from the bottom of the lower central incisors to the top of the upper central

incisors (i.e., from gum line to gum line), while the client continues to hold the bite. This measurement will vary with each client.

**Note:** If the client cannot achieve a natural bite, return to the jaw stability activities.

2. Choose the button (which has already been prepared with the dental floss) of the same size as the measurement taken in 1.
3. Instruct the client to close his/her teeth in a natural bite. Place the flat side of the button against the upper and lower central incisors at midline as pictured in (a). Hold the dental floss in your hand.
4. Instruct the client to close the lips over the button. The button will now be enclosed in the cavity between the closed teeth and the closed lips, as pictured below in (b). Hold this position for 10 seconds, 5 times.

( a )    ( b )

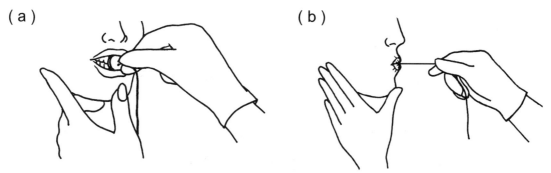

5. Criteria for Success: Once you are sure the client has learned to keep the button in the cavity, pull forward gently with **isometric resistance** as pictured above in (b). Hold for 15 seconds, 5 times.

   Goals:
   1. Practice a natural bite posture
   2. Improve placement for lip mobility
   3. Improve placement for lip closure/rounding
   4. Reduce drooling

   Target Phonemes:
   a. Lip closure phonemes: / m, b, p / and the vocalic / r /
   b. Lip rounding phonemes: / w, o, u, ʊ, ɔ, ʃ(sh), tʃ(ch), dʒ(j) /

Step #2
1. Present a button (with the dental floss attached) that is 1/8" smaller than the original button.
2. Criteria for Success: Repeat the technique described in Step #1. When the client can hold this button between the lips and closed teeth for 15 seconds, 5 times, transition to a 1/8" smaller button.

Goals:

1. Practice a natural bite posture

2. Improve placement for lip mobility

3. Improve placement for lip closure/rounding

4. Reduce drooling

Target Phonemes:

a. Lip closure phonemes: / m, b, p / and the vocalic / r /

b. Lip rounding phonemes: / w,  o, u, ʊ, ɔ, ʃ(sh), ʧ(ch),  ʤ(j) /

Step #3

1. As goals are achieved at each button measurement, reduce the size of the button by 1/8".

2. Criteria for Success:  Continue until the client can hold the 3/8" button in the cavity between the closed lips and the closed teeth for 15 seconds, 5 times.

Goals:

1. Practice a natural bite posture

2. Improve placement for lip mobility

3. Improve placement for lip closure/rounding

4. Reduce drooling

Target Phonemes:

a. Lip closure phonemes: / m, b, p / and the vocalic / r /

b. Lip rounding phonemes: / w,  o, u, ʊ, ɔ, ʃ(sh), ʧ(ch),  ʤ(j) /

# CHEERIO FOR LOWER LIP RETRACTION
## Placement for / f / and / v /

When a client uses a lip closure posture in an attempt to say the phonemes / f / or / v /, the problem may be reduced mobility of the lower lip and jaw-lip dissociation. It will be important to determine if the substitutions of / p / for / f / and / b / for / v / have a placement and movement component. This activity will establish the necessary lower lip retraction placement to support the / f / or / v / at the conversational level.

This activity may be appropriate for clients who make an **auditorially-based standard** / f / but are not using adequate lower lip retraction. An example of this situation is commonly seen with clients who have difficulty learning to produce a standard / r / or standard vocalic / r /. Both of these sounds require tension in the mentalis muscle system. Look at the client as the / f / sound is produced. If the lower lip is not retracting, even slightly, you may have identified why the / r / is not emerging. The standard muscle placement for / f / is the prerequisite movement for / r /.

The specific oral placement or movement goals are listed after each Step.


Suggestions:

1. Once Step #2 of this activity has been mastered, instruct the client to use the upper teeth to remove particles of food from the lower lip at mealtime. Many clients with reduced lower lip retraction use hands or napkins to remove food from the outside of the mouth.

2. You will need Cheerios, Fruit Loops or any other lightweight, similarly shaped food item to implement this activity.
   **Note**: Prior to using any food-based therapy tool, determine if there are allergies or other limiting dietary issues.

3. Safety is always a primary concern when using food-based activities. Make sure the client is capable of chewing and swallowing the Cheerio without choking prior to attempting this activity.

4. Incorporating this technique into a homework plan is easy. First, establish the number of Cheerios that must be removed from the lower lip daily. Then suggest to the parent that the child eat that number of Cheerios per day for breakfast or at snack time, instead of in a bowl with milk as they usually do.
   **Note:** If the Program Plan for this child also includes the Straw Drinking Hierarchy for Thin Liquids, suggest that the child drink the milk through the prescribed therapy straw, thereby accomplishing two homework assignments at one time.

5. Clients who present with saliva control deficits (i.e., drooling) have what I will call a

natural adhesive on the lips already. For those clients who do not have saliva control issues, you will have to decide on which of the following adhesives you feel will be the most beneficial for your client, taking into any identified sensory issues. Possible adhesives include: lip balms, Carmex, water placed on the lower lip with your gloved finger, syrup.

**Note:** Peanut butter should not be used as it may result in a tongue protrusion posture.

6. Prerequisite: "Tongue Depressor for Lip Closure." Complete the Criteria for Success for Step #4 - total 4 pennies.

7. Homework: Establish during the session where the client fails on the hierarchy. Practice that Step at the highest level of successful repetitions for at least one week before moving on to the next level or Step.

Step #1

1. Place a single Cheerio or similar shaped lightweight edible solid at midline on the client's lower lip as pictured below:

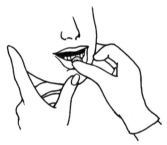

2. Instruct the client to remove the Cheerio into the mouth using the upper teeth as pictured in ( a ).

   **Note:** With some clients you may have to immobilize the upper lip, elevating it slightly with your gloved finger as pictured below in ( b ).

   ( a ) 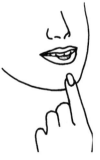    ( b )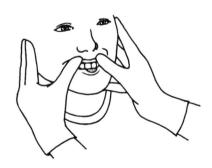

3. <u>Criteria for Success:</u> Remove 5 Cheerios, without a break, by using the upper teeth to make contact with lower lip retraction.

   **Note:** This movement must be independent of assistance to either the upper lip or to the lower jaw.

Goals:

    1. Improve placement for lower lip retraction

    2. Develop jaw-lip dissociation

Target Phonemes:

    a. Lower lip tension/retraction: / f, v /

    b. Lower lip tension/protrusion: / r / and vocalic / r /


## Step #2

1. Repeat the technique described in Step #1.

2. Criteria for Success: Remove 25 Cheerios, without a break, by using the upper teeth to make contact with lower lip retraction.

    Goals:

        1. Improve placement for lower lip retraction

        2. Develop jaw-lip dissociation

    Target Phonemes:

        a. Lower lip tension/retraction: / f, v /

        b. Lower lip tension/protrusion: / r / and vocalic / r /


## Step #3

1. Instruct the client to pretend to remove a Cheerio from the lower lip as practiced above. Monitor to ensure there are no extraneous jaw movements.

2. Criteria for Success: Repeat 1. 50 times, without a break.

    Goals:

        1. Improve placement for lower lip retraction

        2. Develop jaw-lip dissociation

    Target Phonemes:

        a. Lower lip tension/retraction: / f, v /

        b. Lower lip tension/protrusion: / r / and vocalic / r /


## Step #4

1. Continue to work on the standard production of / f or v / in isolation.
   **Note:** Prior to introducing this Step, you will have had to work on auditory awareness and auditory discrimination for your target phoneme.

2. Instruct the client to pretend to remove a Cheerio from the lower lip with the upper teeth. As contact is made, say "freeze."

3. Immediately instruct your client to say the target sound / f or v /, without moving the mouth. After the sound is produced, instruct the client to release the lower lip retraction placement.

4. Repeat the standard production of your target phoneme 50 times or until mastered, as described in 3. before progressing to the word level.

5. Choose any traditional articulation therapy approach you feel comfortable with to work on **carryover**.

Goals:

1. Improve placement for lower lip retraction
2. Develop jaw-lip dissociation.
3. Teach a new muscle memory pattern or motor plan
4. Teach the standard production of / f / and/or /v / in isolation
5. Transition the standard production of / f / and/or /v / into conversational speech

Target Phonemes:

a. Lower lip tension/retraction: / f, v /
b. Lower lip tension/protrusion: / r / and vocalic / r /

# SECTION 3 - TONGUE ACTIVITIES

If there is one single area which has frustrated speech and language pathologists, it is the client who evidences a tongue thrust or too much tongue protrusion at rest and during function: feeding, oral movement and speech sound production. This habitual tongue placement has been associated with clients with low tone (e.g., those with the diagnosis of Down syndrome). It is also seen in the population of cognitively-intact clients who are enrolled in articulation therapy for the correction of the interdental production of sibilant sounds and/or /r/ distortions. As a result of traditional therapy, the client is able to hear the target sound, to identify the target sound in others, and, in some cases, to even say the target sound in isolation or on the single word level using a compensatory posture (i.e., teeth clenching). The client is unable, however, to use the target sound in connected speech, outside of the therapy setting. The reason for this failure to effect carryover has frequently been blamed on the client: the client is not remembering to use the target sound. More often, the reason is the failure of traditional therapy to address the underlying causative factor: insufficient placement and movement skills for tongue grading to support dissociated movement of the lateral margins of the tongue and the tongue-tip.

The activities in this chapter follow the hierarchy of tongue development as was outlined in Chapter 2. Please refer to that hierarchy before introducing any of the following tongue activities.

# RESISTANCE FOR TONGUE BLADE PROTRUSION

## Production Criteria for / θ (th) / and / ð (th) /

Many of you will never use this technique. It is designed for clients who are unable to protrude the tongue between the teeth volitionally. Clients with Cerebral Palsy, Moebius Syndrome or other diagnoses which limit range of motion in the lingual musculature will benefit from this activity. It will improve feeding skills as well as speech clarity. In the past, when a child evidenced a tongue protrusion posture at rest, the approach to teaching that child to keep the tongue within the oral cavity was to push on the tongue-tip. In fact, pushing on the tongue tip encourages protrusion, not retraction. The tongue is the only muscle in the body which has only one insertion. If you push on it, it will push back towards you.

This activity is designed to increase awareness, placement, mobility and muscle memory for dissociated tongue protrusion. At the conclusion of "Resistance for Tongue Blade Protrusion," you will be ready to teach the tongue protrusion phonemes / θ (th) / and / ð (th) /. In addition to targeting the / θ (th) / and / ð (th) /, this activity should be used if the client with whom you are working is retracting the tongue during speech sound production. One of the primary causes for a lateral production of sibilant sounds is too much tongue retraction. Standard sibilants are made with a combination of graded tongue movements. The back of the tongue is retracted for stability, the sides are spread and the tip of the tongue is tightened. You will need to do this activity before you can address the tongue-tip component.

The specific placement or movement goals are listed after each Step.

Suggestions:

1. If you are using this activity to remediate the lateral production of sibilant sounds, upon its completion progress to the activity entitled, "Tongue-Tip Lateralization."
   **Note:** Whenever you are working on any component of tongue grading, you should be using the activity entitled, "Straw Drinking Hierarchy."
2. Use a tight-fitting glove for this exercise to protect the child as well as yourself.
   **Note:** Refer to the information concerning how to choose the most appropriate glove type and size described in the activity entitled, "Crumbs."
3. You may use any of the following therapy tools to implement this activity:
   a. Gloved pointer finger
   b. NUK massager
   c. Ice pop/Ice finger
   d. Highly-flavored, firm licorice stick
   e. TOOTHETTE®: non-flavored or dipped into a favorite flavor

4. This technique can be used with clients who have minimal cognitive awareness, as the technique is based on a stimulus-response model.

5. Homework: Establish during the session where the client fails on the hierarchy. Practice that Step at the highest level of successful repetitions for at least one week before moving onto the next level or Step.

Step#1

1. Instruct the client to open his/her mouth. You may demonstrate or assist in mouth opening for cognitively or severely motor-impaired clients.

2. Use your gloved, pointed index finger, or one of the other suggested therapy tools, to push firmly on the tongue tip until the blade is retracted into the oral cavity. Release quickly and wait for a response.

   **Note:** An acceptable response will be any movement within the lingual musculature following the removal of the therapy tool, excluding the passive repositioning of the muscles.

3. Criteria for Success:  Repeat this technique 10 times or until the client refuses the intervention.

   **Note:** Whenever appropriate, it is important to use verbal explanations to describe to the client what he/she is "feeling" in the tongue musculature.  You may use a mirror to reinforce volitional movement in response to the pushing on the tongue-tip (resistance therapy).

   Goals:
      1. Increase awareness of the tongue
      2. Improve range of motion in the tongue
      3. Teach placement for tongue protrusion

   Target Phonemes:
      a. Tongue-tip: / t, d, l, n, k, g, s, z, ʃ(sh), ʧ(ch), ʤ(j) /
      b. Tongue Protrusion: / θ (th) / and / ð (th) /

Step #2

1. Repeat the technique described in Step #1 one time.  As you remove the tool, instruct the client: "Stick out your tongue."

2. Criteria for Success:  When the client consistently demonstrates even a minimal tongue forward protrusion in response to the push, 10 times, progress to Step #3.

161

Goals:

1. Increase awareness of the tongue
2. Improve range of motion and grading in the lingual musculature
3. Stimulate tongue protrusion
4. Teach placement for volitional tongue protrusion
5. Improve jaw-tongue dissociation

Target Phonemes:

a. Tongue-tip: / t, d, l, n, k, g, s, z, ʃ(sh), ʧ(ch), ʤ(j) /
b. Tongue Protrusion: / θ (th) / and / ð (th) /

## Step #3

1. Repeat the technique described in Step #1 one time. As you remove the tool, instruct the client: "Stick out your tongue." Wait for a response.

2. Touch the tongue tip lightly with the tool. As you remove the tool, instruct the client: "Stick out your tongue." Wait for the response of even minimal tongue forward protrusion in response to the light touch, one time.

3. Criteria for Success: Alternate between 1. and 2. of this Step to achieve one unit (10 times).

   **Note:** A response must be seen after each stimuli to consider the unit completed.

   Goals:

   1. Increase awareness of the tongue
   2. Improve range of motion and grading in the lingual musculature
   3. Stimulate tongue protrusion
   4. Teach placement for volitional tongue protrusion
   5. Improve jaw-tongue dissociation

   Target Phonemes:

   a. Tongue-tip: / t, d, l, n, k, g, s, z, ʃ(sh), ʧ(ch), ʤ(j) /
   b. Tongue Protrusion: / θ (th) / and / ð (th) /

## Step #4

1. Instruct the client: "Stick out your tongue." Wait for a forward tongue movement. Reinforce verbally and with a mirror, one time.

2. Instruct the client to make a funny face. This instruction should result in releasing the tongue protrusion placement, one time.

162

3.  <u>Criteria for Success:</u>  Alternate between 1. and 2. of this step 10 times, or until you are sure volitional tongue protrusion placement has been mastered.

    <u>Goals:</u>

    1.  Increase awareness of the tongue
    2.  Improve range of motion and grading in the lingual musculature
    3.  Stimulate tongue protrusion
    4.  Teach placement for volitional tongue protrusion
    5.  Improve jaw-tongue dissociation

    <u>Target Phonemes:</u>

    a.  Tongue-tip: / t, d, l, n, k, g, s, z, ʃ(sh), ʧ(ch), ʤ(j) /
    b.  Tongue Protrusion:  / θ (th) / and / ð (th) /

## Step #5

1.  Instruct the client: "Stick out your tongue," and then to release that position, 50 times.
2.  Introduce the standard production of / θ (th) / and / ð (th) / in isolation.

    **Note:** Prior to introducing this Step, you will have had to work on auditory awareness and auditory discrimination for your target phoneme.

3.  Instruct the client to stick his/her tongue-tip out until it is slightly protruded between the teeth.  Have the client hold that placement to say / θ (th) / or / ð (th) /.
4.  <u>Criteria for Success:</u>  Repeat the standard production of your target phoneme, 50 times or until mastered, before progressing to the word level.

    <u>Goals:</u>

    1.  Increase awareness of the tongue
    2.  Improve range of motion and grading in the lingual musculature
    3.  Stimulate tongue protrusion
    4.  Teach placement for volitional tongue protrusion
    5.  Improve jaw-tongue dissociation

    <u>Target Phonemes:</u>

    a.  Tongue-tip: / t, d, l, n, k, g, s, z,  ʃ(sh), ʧ(ch), ʤ(j) /
    b.  Tongue Protrusion:  / θ (th) / and / ð (th) /

# TONGUE BLADE RETRACTION - Summary

Any lip protrusion activity will encourage tongue retraction. The following activities (which have been described previously) should also be used to address placement for tongue blade retraction and grading:

1. **Straw Drinking Hierarchy**: Refer to the complete explanation of this technique in this book. Most clients will begin this technique with Straw #1.

   **Note:** Refer to the video, *Straws as Therapy Tools*, for a complete explanation of the technique for yourself, parents or teachers.

2. **Horn Blowing Hierarchy**: Refer to the complete explanation of this technique in this book.

   a. Lower-functioning clients will begin this technique with Horn #1.

   b. Higher-functioning clients with interdental production of sibilant sounds as the only speech clarity deficits, may begin this hierarchy with Horn #9. Horns #9 through #12 directly address placement for tongue retraction.

   **Note:** Refer to the video, *Horns as Therapy Tools*, for a complete explanation of the technique for yourself, parents or teachers.

3. **Bubble Blowing Hierarchy**: Refer to the complete explanation of this technique in this book

   a. Lower-functioning clients will begin this technique with Step #1.

   b. Higher-functioning clients, with interdental production of sibilant sounds as the only speech clarity deficits, may begin this hierarchy with Step #6 through #8 which directly address placement for tongue retraction.

   **Note:** Refer to the video, *Bubbles as Therapy Tools*, for a complete explanation of the technique for yourself, parents or teachers.

4. **Golf Ball Air Hockey**: Refer to the complete explanation of this technique in this book.

# TONGUE BLADE RETRACTION WITH RESISTANCE

Since we know pushing on the tongue blade will encourage protrusion, conversely, pulling on the tongue blade will teach retraction. Resistance therapy has proven to be very beneficial for teaching volitional retraction of the tongue blade. Use this activity with clients who can understand the verbal direction of "Pull your tongue back into your mouth."

The specific oral placement and movement goals are listed after each Step.

Suggestions:
1. You will need a thin washcloth, a cotton handkerchief or gauze to implement this a activity.
2. Do not "pull out" or hold the tongue tightly, as it will inhibit the client's ability to perform this activity.
3. Homework: Establish during the session where the client fails on the hierarchy. Practice that Step at the highest level of successful repetitions for at least one week before moving onto the next level or Step.

Step #1
1. Instruct the client to stick out his/her tongue. You do not need a pointed tongue to teach this activity.
2. Fold the cloth/gauze into a 5" x 1" strip. Begin on the underside of the tongue and wrap the cloth/gauze around the front of the tongue, as pictured below:

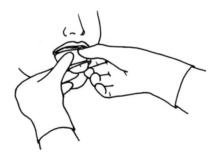

3. Once the cloth/gauze is in place, hold no more firmly than is required to stabilize the protruded tongue. Do not squeeze or pull on the tongue.
4. Instruct the client: "Pull your tongue back into your mouth," as you maintain slight resistance with the cloth/gauze.
   **Note:** Monitor to ensure the client is using tongue retraction and not the compensatory pattern of whole body or head retraction to remove the tongue from the cloth/gauze.

5. <u>Criteria for Success:</u> Repeat this technique 10 times before progressing to Step #2.

    <u>Goals:</u>

    1. Teach volitional tongue retraction

    2. Teach jaw-tongue dissociation

    <u>Target Phonemes:</u>

    All phonemes in English with the exception of: / θ (th) / and / ð (th) /

<u>Step #2</u>

1. Repeat the technique described in Step #1 with slightly more resistance.

2. <u>Criteria for Success:</u> Work up to 15 repetitions, before progressing to Step #3.

    **Note:** Remember to use resistance only. Do not pull the tongue out.

    <u>Goals:</u>

    1. Teach volitional tongue retraction

    2. Teach jaw-tongue dissociation

    <u>Target Phonemes:</u>

    All phonemes in English with the exception of: / θ (th) / and / ð (th) /

<u>Step #3</u>

1. Instruct the client: "Pull your tongue back into your mouth." Wait for a tongue retraction movement. Reinforce verbally and with a mirror.

2. Instruct the client to make a funny face. This instruction should result in the release of the tongue retraction placement, 1 time.

3. <u>Criteria for Success:</u> Alternate between 1. and 2. of this step 10 times, or until you are sure placement for volitional tongue retraction has been mastered.

    <u>Goals:</u>

    1. Teach volitional tongue retraction

    2. Teach jaw-tongue dissociation

    <u>Target Phonemes:</u>

    All phonemes in English with the exception of: / θ (th) / and / ð (th) /

# TONGUE-TIP LATERALIZATION (The jaw must be stable.)

In order to successfully complete the following activity, the client must have sufficient tongue blade retraction to support the development of true **lateralization** within the oral cavity. By definition, true lateralization occurs when the tongue-tip touches the lower back molar on alternating sides of the mouth without associated jaw movement. In the case of a client without molars, the tongue position would be the same. For those of you who are testing lateralization with the tongue protruded, you are missing a critical component of lateralization: **retraction**.

It is important to understand another component of tongue-tip lateralization: movement is based upon sensation. For example, when you brush your teeth, note what happens to your tongue-tip. In most cases, the stimulation of brushing the teeth/gums results in the lateralization of the tongue-tip to that spot. In others, the tongue-tip moves away from the stimuli. In both cases, the tongue-tip lateralizes in response to the awareness of touch. This knowledge is critical to the success of the following techniques.

The same scenario is noted when we eat. We find the tongue-tip lateralizes to the lower back molar ridge when we place food in that area. We also note that to move food from the back molars we use our tongue-tip. Therefore, in addition to working on the following activity for tongue-tip lateralization, it is beneficial to teach the client to bite and chew on the back molars or back molar ridges to stimulate tongue-tip lateralization.

An inability to lateralize the tongue-tip to the lower back molar on alternating sides of the mouth may be secondary to: muscle weakness, insufficient jaw-tongue dissociation, motor-planning deficits or a frenum that is too short to allow the tongue-tip to reach the back molar or molar ridge. The possibility of structural deficits should be evaluated prior to the introduction of these techniques.

Remember, in a developmental hierarchy, tongue-tip lateralization is first achieved from **midline** to either side. When the control and movement from midline to one side then from midline to the other side is sufficient, the tongue-tip will lateralize across midline. The following activity is divided into two sections:

Section 1: Tongue-Tip Lateralization - Midline to Either Side

Section 2: Tongue-Tip Lateralization - Across Midline

In most cases, after "Midline to Either Side" is mastered through placement activities and during feeding, the tongue naturally learns to move across midline. In other words, the mobility of the lateral muscles on both sides of the tongue is sufficient to move the tongue-tip to the lower back molar or molar ridge on alternating sides of the mouth. If this is the case with your client, you will not have to work on Section 2: Tongue-Tip Lateralization - Across Midline. For those of you working with clients who do not make this transition spontaneously (e.g., clients with Agenesis of the Corpus Collusum), Section 2: "Tongue-Tip Lateralization - Across Midline" will teach the movement.

The specific oral placement and movement goals are listed after each Step.

Suggestions:
1. When using food items for this activity (e.g., therapy tools: **highly flavored licorice, Laffy Taffy**), make sure the therapy tool is very hard. The purpose of this activity is to bite down on a hard surface to stabilize the jaw so the tongue-tip can dissociate for independent lateralization. If the client can bite through the therapy tool, it should not be used. Highly flavored licorice can be hardened by leaving it outside of the package for a few days. Laffy Taffy can be hardened by keeping it in the refrigerator.
2. Other therapy tools that have been used successfully to implement this activity include: TalkTools® Jaw Grading Bite Blocks, ARK's Probe, and Slim Jim Sticks. The therapy tool has to be wide enough to allow you to see what is happening inside of the mouth after the bite is achieved.
3. Homework: Establish during the session where the client fails on the hierarchy. Practice that Step at the highest level of successful repetitions for at least one week before moving on to the next level or Step.

**Section 1: Tongue-Tip Lateralization - Midline to Either Side**

Step #1
1. Instruct the client to open his/her mouth.
2. Place the tip of the therapy tool (suggestions above) on the surface of the lower back molar, on the left side, extending from the side of the mouth, as pictured below.

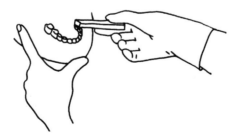

3. Instruct the client to bite down on, but not through, the therapy tool. A **natural bite** is mandatory for this activity.

**Note:** If a natural bite cannot be achieved despite numerous attempts using

**assisted jaw stability**, return to the jaw stability activities before attempting this activity.
4. While maintaining a natural bite, instruct the client to touch the tip of the therapy tool with the tongue-tip.
5. Instruct the client to open his/her mouth as you remove the therapy tool.
6. Criteria for Success: Repeat this Step 5 times before progressing to Step #2.

Goals:
1. Establish a natural bite
2. Stabilize tongue retraction
3. Teach placement for tongue-tip lateralization from midline to the left side of the mouth
4. Develop jaw-tongue dissociation

Target Phonemes: A prerequisite for establishing stability in the tongue for the development of standard co-articulation of all speech sounds

Step #2
1. Instruct the client to open his/her mouth.
2. Place the tip of the therapy tool on the surface of the lower back molar, on the right side, extending from the side of the mouth, as pictured below.

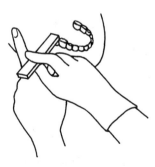

3. Instruct the client to bite down on, but not through, the therapy tool. A natural bite is mandatory for this activity.
   **Note:** If a natural bite cannot be achieved despite numerous attempts using **assisted jaw stability**, return to the jaw stability activities before attempting this activity.
4. While maintaining a natural bite, instruct the client to touch the tip of the therapy tool with the tongue-tip.
5. Instruct the client to open his/her mouth as you remove the therapy tool.
6. Criteria for Success: Repeat this Step 5 times before progressing to Step #3.

Goals:

1. Establish a natural bite
2. Stabilize tongue retraction
3. Teach placement for tongue-tip lateralization from midline to the right side of the mouth
4. Develop jaw-tongue dissociation

Target Phonemes: A prerequisite for establishing stability in the tongue for the development of standard co-articulation of all speech sounds

Step #3

1. Instruct the client to open his/her mouth.
2. Place the tip of the therapy tool on the surface of the lower back molar, on the left side, extending from the side of the mouth, as pictured in Step #1.
3. Instruct the client to bite down on, but not through, the therapy tool.
4. While maintaining a natural bite, instruct the client to touch the tip of the therapy tool with the tongue-tip. Open the mouth and repeat on the right side (1 unit).
5. Criteria for Success: Repeat 4. in this step 10 times before progressing to Step #4.
**Note:** Monitor to ensure the jaw remains stable throughout the repetitions.

Goals:

1. Establish a natural bite
2. Stabilize tongue retraction
3. Teach placement for tongue-tip lateralization from midline to the left side of the mouth and tongue-tip from midline to the right side of the mouth
4. Develop jaw-tongue dissociation

Target Phonemes: A prerequisite for establishing stability in the tongue for the development of standard co-articulation of all speech sounds

Step #4

1. Instruct the client to open his/her mouth.
2. Place the tip of the therapy tool on the surface of the lower back molar, on the left side, extending from the side of the mouth.
3. Instruct the client to bite down, but not through, the therapy tool.
4. While maintaining a natural bite, instruct the client to touch the tip of the therapy tool using the tongue-tip using three rapid movements (tickle). Repeat on the right side of the mouth (1 unit).

170

5. <u>Criteria for Success:</u> Repeat 4. in this step 10 times before progressing to Section 2: Tongue-Tip Lateralization Across Midline."

**Note:** Monitor to ensure the jaw remains stable throughout the repetitions.

Goals:
1. Establish a natural bite
2. Stabilize tongue retraction
3. Teach placement for tongue-tip lateralization from midline to the left side of the mouth and tongue-tip from midline to the right side of the mouth
4. Develop jaw-tongue dissociation

<u>Target Phonemes:</u> A prerequisite for establishing stability in the tongue for the development of standard co-articulation of all speech sounds

## Section 2: Tongue-Tip Lateralization Across Midline

<u>Step #1</u>
1. In Steps #1 through #3 you will use the activity entitled: "5-Position Bite."
2. Instruct the client to open his/her mouth.
3. Place the tip of the therapy tool on the surface of the lower back molar, on the right side of the mouth, as pictured below at position "a."

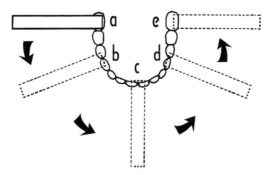

4. Instruct the client to bite down on, but not through, the therapy tool and to then to touch the tip of the therapy tool with the tongue-tip. Once the touch is complete, open the mouth and remove the therapy tool.
5. Immediately place the tip of the therapy tool on the surface of the tooth at position "b." Repeat the "Bite-Touch-Release" instruction.
6. Immediately place the tip of the therapy tool on the surface of the tooth at position "c." Repeat the "Bite-Touch-Release" instruction.
7. Immediately place the tip of the therapy tool on the surface of the tooth at position "d." Repeat the "Bite-Touch-Release" instruction.

8. Immediately place the tip of the therapy tool on the surface of the tooth at position "e." Repeat the "Bite-Touch-Release" instruction.

   **Note:** If done correctly, this will teach the tongue-tip to move across midline while the jaw remains still.

9. Criteria for Success: Repeat this Step 5 times successfully.

   Goals:

   1. Stabilize tongue retraction
   2. Teach placement for tongue-tip lateralization across midline from right to left
   3. Develop jaw-tongue dissociation

   Target Phonemes: A prerequisite for establishing stability in the tongue for the development of standard co-articulation of all speech sounds


Step #2

1. Repeat Step #1 working from the left side of the mouth to the right side of the mouth.

2. Criteria for Success: Repeat this Step 5 times successfully.

   Goals:

   1. Stabilize tongue retraction
   2. Teach placement for tongue-tip lateralization across midline from left to right
   3. Develop jaw-tongue dissociation

   Target Phonemes: A prerequisite for establishing stability in the tongue for the development of standard co-articulation of all speech sounds


Step #3

1. Repeat the technique described in Steps #1 and #2, working from left to right, 1 time, immediately followed by working from right to left, 1 time (1 unit).

2. Criteria for Success: Repeat this Step 5 times successfully.

   Goals:

   1. Stabilize tongue retraction
   2. Teach placement for tongue-tip lateralization across midline in both directions.
   3. Develop jaw-tongue dissociation

   Target Phonemes: A prerequisite for establishing stability in the tongue for the development of standard co-articulation of all speech sounds

## Step #4

1. Use a firm, textured cube of food for this Step. Cut the cube into the size of a Cheerio.

2. Place the cube on the surface of the lower back molar, on the left side of the mouth, with your gloved fingers. Remove your hand.

3. Instruct the client to move the cube to the surface of the lower back molar, on the right side of the mouth, with the mouth open slightly and with minimal jaw movement.

   **Note:** If the jaw slides or moves excessively or if the client attempts to use gravity to move the cube of food, return to the jaw stability activities.

4. <u>Criteria for Success:</u> Repeat this Step 5 times successfully.

   <u>Goals:</u>

   1. Stabilize tongue retraction
   2. Improve placement for tongue-tip lateralization strength across midline from left to right
   3. Develop jaw-tongue dissociation.

   <u>Target Phonemes:</u> A prerequisite for establishing stability in the tongue for the development of standard co-articulation of all speech sounds

## Step #5

1. Use a firm, textured cube of food for this Step. Cut the cube into the size of a Cheerio.

2. Place the cube on the surface of the lower back molar, on the right side of the mouth, with your gloved fingers. Remove your hand.

3. Instruct the client to move the cube to the surface of the lower back molar, on the left side of the mouth, with the mouth open slightly and with minimal jaw movement.

   **Note:** If the jaw slides or moves excessively or if the client attempts to use gravity to move the cube of food, return to the jaw stability activities.

4. <u>Criteria for Success:</u> Repeat this Step 5 times successfully.

   <u>Goals:</u>

   1. Stabilize tongue retraction
   2. Improve placement for tongue-tip lateralization strength across midline from right to left
   3. Develop jaw-tongue dissociation

   <u>Target Phonemes:</u> A prerequisite for establishing stability in the tongue for the development of standard co-articulation of all speech sounds

## Step # 6

1.  Place a Cheerio-sized cube on the surface of the lower back molar, on the left side of the client's mouth, with your gloved fingers.

2.  Instruct the client to move the cube to the surface of the lower back molar, on the right side of the mouth, then immediately move it back to the surface of the lower back molar on the left side of the mouth, with the mouth open slightly and with minimal jaw movement (1 unit).

3.  Criteria for Success: Repeat this Step 10 times successfully.

    **Note:** Monitor to ensure the jaw remains stable throughout the repetitions.

    Goals:

    1.  Stabilize tongue retraction
    2.  Improve placement for tongue-tip lateralization across midline in both directions
    3.  Develop jaw-tongue dissociation

    Target Phonemes: A prerequisite for establishing stability in the tongue for the development of standard co-articulation of all speech sounds

    **Note:** The TalkTools® Tongue-Tip Lateralization Tool can also be used to teach tongue-tip lateralization from midline to side and across midline.

# TONGUE-TIP POINTING

In general, when tongue-tip lateralization to the back molar on alternating sides of the mouth has developed, a tongue-tip point is achieved that can be used to teach tip elevation and depression. With some clients, however, tongue tip mobility is reduced. Clients with Cerebral Palsy frequently have difficulty achieving dissociated tongue-tip movement. Using massage on the lateral margins of the tongue will help to establish the tip.

The specific oral placement and movement goals are listed after each Step.

Suggestions:

1. You may use any of the following items to implement this activity: a highly-flavored licorice stick, a NUK massager, an ARK's Probe, an ice finger, an Ice Stick, a TOOTHETTE® a Slim Jim stick.

2. This technique should not be given for homework. Instead, it should be used to stimulate a tongue-tip point in the therapy room which can then be used actively in a tongue-tip elevation or depression activity.

Step #1

1. Instruct the client to open his/her mouth and to stick out the tongue. If the client cannot protrude the tongue, return to the tongue blade protrusion activities.

2. Place the massager along the lateral margin of the tongue on the left side. Use the massager to stimulate the sides of the tongue from posterior to anterior.

3. Criteria for Success: Work in units of 3 rapid movements on the left side followed immediately by 3 rapid movements on the right side (1 unit), 3 times.
   Goal: Improve placement for tongue-tip pointing
   Target Phonemes: / t, d, l, n, k, g, s, z, ʃ(sh), ʧ(ch), ʤ(j) /

Step #2

1. Repeat the technique described in Step #1 using only 2 rapid movements from posterior to anterior on alternating sides of the tongue.

2. Criteria for Success: When a tongue-tip point is achieved 5 times in direct response to this stimulation, transition the tongue-tip point immediately to a tongue-tip activity.
   Goal: Improve placement for tongue-tip pointing
   Target Phonemes: / t, d, l, n, k, g, s, z, ʃ(sh), ʧ(ch), ʤ(j) /

175

## CHEERIO FOR TONGUE-TIP ELEVATION Production Criteria for / t, d, n, l /

This activity is designed to increase awareness, placement, mobility and muscle memory for tongue-tip elevation. At the conclusion of this activity teach the tongue-tip elevation phonemes / t, d, n, l, ʃ(sh), tʃ(ch), ʤ(j)/

**Note:** For many clients, tongue-tip elevation will be the placement for the standard production of / s, z /.

The specific oral placement and movement goals are listed after each Step.

Suggestions:

1. If the client is unable to achieve or create a tongue-tip, do not attempt this activity. Choose one of the following activities instead, to determine where on the **Tongue Grading Hierarchy** your client is functioning:

    a. "Resistance for Tongue Blade Protrusion"

    b. "Tongue Blade Retraction"

    c. "Blade Retraction with Resistance"

    d. "Tongue-Tip Lateralization"

    e. "Tongue-Tip Pointing"

2. You may use any of the following tools to implement this activity: Cheerio, Fruit Loop, orthodontic rubber band.

3. The prerequisite tongue movement for tongue-tip elevation is tongue-tip lateralization. The client, therefore, should have no difficulty moving the Cheerio to the molar surface for safe chewing. If, however, the client cannot lateralize the tongue-tip to move the Cheerio, you are attempting this technique too soon. Return to the tongue lateralization activities.

4. If the client is unable to perform this task without elevating the jaw to assist in the tongue-tip elevation despite numerous attempts, return to the jaw stability activities.

5. If the sides or front of the tongue protrude, return to the tongue retraction activities.

6. Before introducing Step #4 in this activity, you will have to work on the auditory awareness and auditory discrimination skills for the target phonemes / t, d, n, **or** l / . The client must know when and where to produce the target phoneme, through traditional articulation therapy, prior to the introduction of Step #4. Carryover into the word level and into conversational speech will then move rapidly.

7. Homework: Establish during the session where the client fails on the hierarchy. Practice that Step at the highest level of successful repetitions for at least one week before moving on to the next level or Step.

176

## Step #1

1. Instruct the client to open his/her mouth to a medium-to-low jaw height. To ensure proper position, place your thumb on the client's chin and pull down gently.
   **Note:** For a complete explanation refer to the Jaw Height Hierarchy described in this book.
2. Place the Cheerio on the alveolar ridge with your gloved finger as pictured in (a) below.
3. Instruct the client to put his/her tongue-tip in the hole of the Cheerio.
4. Once the tongue-tip is in the hole of the Cheerio, remove your finger.
5. Release your thumb from the client's chin as pictured below in ( b ).

( a )            ( b )

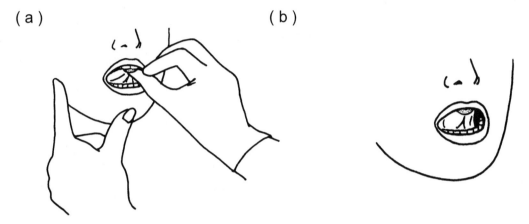

6. Criteria for Success: Instruct the client to keep the his/her jaw open and to hold the tongue-tip in the Cheerio hole for 5 seconds. When this goal is achieved, tell the client: "Eat it." Repeat this task 5 times (1 unit).
   **Note:** Indicate the unit has been completed by filling in the first box in the chart on the next page with a sticker, stamp or color it with a crayon.
   
   Goals:
   1. Improve placement for tongue-tip elevation
   2. Develop jaw-tongue dissociation
   
   Target Phonemes:  / t, d, l, n, s, z, ʃ(sh), tʃ(ch), dʒ(j) /

Step #2

1. Repeat the technique described in Step #1.
2. Continue to fill in the chart on the previous page as each target number is achieved. Each box in the chart represents 5 Cheerio trials (1 unit) at the specific number of seconds written inside the box.
3. Criteria for Success: When you finish the chart, the client will be able to hold his/her elevated tongue-tip in the hole of the Cheerio for 50 seconds, 5 times.

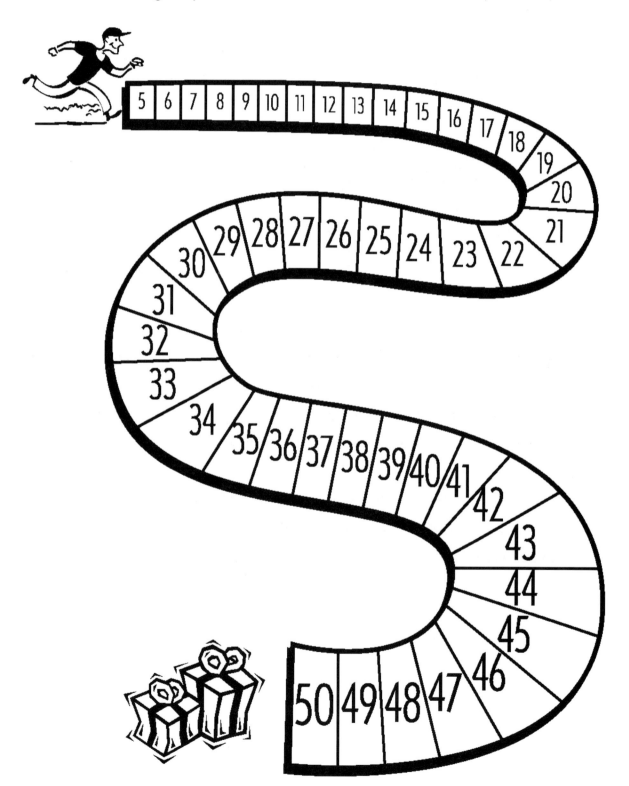

178

Goals:

1. Improve placement for tongue-tip elevation
2. Develop jaw-tongue dissociation

Target Phonemes: / t, d, l, n, s, z, ʃ(sh), tʃ(ch), ʤ(j) /

## Step #3

1. Instruct the client: "Open your mouth and put your tongue-tip where the Cheerio was." Hold that position for 1 second and then release it (muscle memory).

2. Criteria for Success: Repeat #1, 50 times. Make sure the jaw remains stationary during this entire activity.

   Goals:

   1. Improve placement for tongue-tip elevation
   2. Develop jaw-tongue dissociation
   3. Teach a new motor plan

   Target Phonemes: / t, d, l, n, s, z, ʃ(sh), tʃ(ch), ʤ(j) /

## Step #4

1. At this point, you are ready to introduce the standard production of: / t, d, n or l / in isolation.

   **Note:** Prior to introducing this Step, you will have had to work on auditory awareness and auditory discrimination for your target phoneme.

2. Instruct the client to put his/her tongue-tip up where the Cheerio was and then to say either "t," "d," "n," or "l." Make sure the tongue-tip moves away from the alveolar ridge after the production of the sound in isolation.

   **Note:** When working with a client with motor planning difficulties, apraxia or dyspraxia, the Cheerio may have to be used initially in association with the production of the target phoneme to assist in motor planning. It may also be used in conjunction with direct speech intervention. The Cheerio must be eliminated before progressing to 3.

3. Repeat the standard production of your target phoneme 50 times or until mastered in isolation before progressing onto the word level.

4. Choose any traditional articulation therapy approach you feel comfortable with to work on **carryover**.

Goals:

1. Improve placement for tongue-tip elevation

2. Develop jaw-tongue dissociation

3. Teach the standard production of: / t, d, n, or l / in isolation

4. Transition the standard production of: / t, d, n, or l / into conversational speech

Target Phonemes: / t, d, l, n /

**Note:** The TalkTools® Tongue-Tip Elevation-Depression Tool can also be used to teach tongue-tip elevation.

# CHEERIO FOR TONGUE-TIP DEPRESSION   Production Criteria for / k, g /

This activity is designed to increase awareness, placement, mobility and muscle memory for tongue-tip depression. At the conclusion of this activity you can teach the tongue-tip depression phonemes / k, g /.

> **Note:** Tongue-tip depression is necessary for the standard production of:
> / k, g /. For many clients it will be the placement for the standard production of
> / s, z /. The specific oral placement and movement goals are listed after each Step.

Suggestions:

1. If the client is unable to achieve or create a tongue-tip, do not attempt this activity. Instead, return to the activity entitled, "Tongue-Tip Pointing," described in this book.

2. You may use any of the following tools to implement this exercise: Cheerio, Fruit Loop, orthodontic rubber band.

3. If the client is unable to perform this task without sliding or jutting the jaw to assist in the tongue-tip depression despite numerous attempts, return to the jaw stability activities.

4. The prerequisite tongue movement for dissociated tongue-tip depression is tongue-tip lateralization. The client, therefore, should have no difficulty moving the Cheerio to the molar surface for safe chewing. If, however, the client cannot lateralize the tongue tip to move the Cheerio, you are attempting this technique too soon. Return to the activity entitled, "Tongue-Tip Lateralization."

5. If the sides or front of the tongue protrude, return to the activity entitled, "Tongue Blade Retraction."

6. Before introducing Step #4 in this activity, you will have to work on the auditory awareness and auditory discrimination skills for the target phonemes / k, g /. The client must know when and where to produce the target phoneme, through traditional articulation therapy, prior to the introduction of Step #4. Carryover into the word level and into conversational speech will then move rapidly.

7. Homework: Establish during the session where the client fails on the hierarchy. Practice that Step at the highest level of successful repetitions for at least one week before moving on to the next level or Step.

Step #1

1. Instruct the client to open his/her mouth to a medium jaw height. To ensure proper position, place your thumb on the client's chin and pull down gently.

**Note:** For a complete explanation refer to the **Jaw Height Hierarchy**, described in this book.

2. Place the Cheerio at midline on the lower gum ridge with your gloved finger.
3. Instruct the client to put the tongue-tip in the hole of the Cheerio, as pictured below.

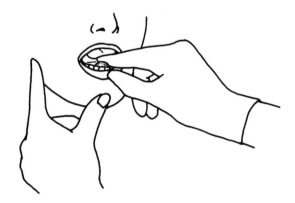

4. Once the tongue-tip is in the hole of the Cheerio, remove your finger.
5. Criteria for Success: Instruct the client to keep the jaw open and hold the tongue-tip in the Cheerio hole for 5 seconds. When the time goal is achieved, tell the client, "Eat it." Repeat this task 5 times (1 unit).

**Note:** Indicate that the unit has been completed by filling in the first box in the chart below with a sticker, stamp, or color it with a crayon.

Goals:
   1. Improve placement for tongue-tip depression
   2. Develop jaw-tongue dissociation

Target Phonemes: / k, g, s, z /

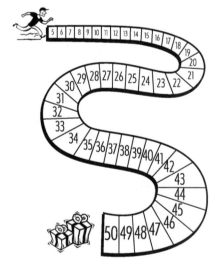

Step #2
1. Repeat the technique described in Step #1.
2. Continue to fill in the chart as each target number is achieved. Each box in the chart represents 5 Cheerio trials (1 unit) at the specific number of seconds written inside the box.
3. Criteria for Success: When you finish the chart the client will be able to hold the depressed tongue-tip in the hole of the Cheerio for 50 seconds, 5 times.

Goals:

1.  Improve placement for tongue-tip depression

2.  Develop jaw-tongue dissociation.

Target Phonemes: / k, g, s, z /


## Step #3

1.  Instruct the client: "Put your tongue-tip where the Cheerio was." Hold that position for 1 second and then release it (muscle memory).

2.  Criteria for Success: Repeat #1, 50 times. Make sure the jaw remains stationary during this entire activity.

    Goals:

    1.  Improve placement for tongue-tip depression

    2.  Develop jaw-tongue dissociation

    3.  Teach a new muscle memory pattern

    Target Phonemes: / k, g, s, z /


## Step #4

1.  Introduce the standard production of: / k or g / in isolation.
    **Note:** Remember prior to introducing this Step, you will have had to work on auditory awareness and auditory discrimination for your target phoneme.

2.  Instruct the client to put the tongue-tip down where the Cheerio was and to then say either / k / or / g /. Make sure the tongue-tip moves away from the gum ridge after the production of the sound in isolation.
    **Note:** When working with a client with motor planning difficulties, apraxia or dyspraxia, the Cheerio may have to be used initially in association with the production of the target phoneme to assist in motor planning. The Cheerio must be eliminated before progressing to 3.

3.  Criteria for Success: Repeat the standard production of your target phoneme 50 times or until mastered in isolation before progressing to the word level.

4.  Choose any traditional articulation therapy approach with which you feel comfortable to work on carryover.

    Goals:

    1.  Improve placement for tongue-tip depression

    2.  Develop jaw-tongue dissociation

183

3. Teach placement for the standard production of: / k or g / in isolation

4. Transition placement for the standard production of: / k or g / into conversational speech

<u>Target Phonemes:</u> / k, g /

**Note:** The TalkTools® Tongue-Tip Elevation-Depression Tool can be used to teach tongue-tip depression.

**TONGUE-TIP UP AND DOWN**     **Production Criteria for / s-z /**

Once placement for dissociated tongue-tip elevation and tongue-tip depression are mastered, it will be important to teach co-articulation of these movements. Otherwise, clients may develop a speech pattern where the tongue-tip is "fixed" in either the "tongue-tip up" position or in the "tongue-tip down" position.

This activity is designed to increase awareness, placement, movement and muscle memory for tongue-tip mobility. At the conclusion of this activity, you will be ready to teach the phonemes / s, z / in either the tongue-tip elevation or tongue-tip depression position.

The specific oral placement and movement goals are listed after each Step.

Suggestions:

1.  If the client is unable to perform the task described in this activity without sliding or jutting the jaw to assist in the tongue-tip elevation or in the tongue-tip depression despite numerous attempts, return to the jaw stability activities.

2.  If the client's tongue protrudes interdentally at any time during the practicing of this activity, you should identify the deficit:

    a.  If there is too much blade protrusion, return to the "Tongue Blade Retraction" activity.

    b.  If the tip does not elevate and depress with speed, return to the "Tongue-Tip Elevation" activity and then on to the "Tongue-Tip Depression" activity.

3.  You will need one tongue depressor to implement this activity.

4.  Homework: Establish during the session where the client fails on the hierarchy. Practice that Step at the highest level of successful repetitions for at least one week before moving on to the next level or Step.

Step #1

1.  Instruct the client to open his/her mouth to a medium height.

2.  Criteria for Success:

    a.  While maintaining that jaw height, instruct the client: "Put your tongue-tip up, where it was for the Cheerio." Hold this position for 1 second.

    b.  Instruct the client: "Put your tongue-tip down, where it was for the Cheerio, without moving your jaw." Hold this position for 1 second (a. + b. = 1 unit) 1 time.

185

Goals:

1. Develop jaw-tongue dissociation
2. Teach placement for dissociated tongue-tip elevation and depression as a component of mobility and agility during co-articulation

Target Phonemes:

/ t, d, n, l, s, z, ʃ(sh), ʧ(ch), ʤ(j) /in conjunction with all vowels

## Step #2

1. While maintaining a medium jaw height, hold for 1 second and then immediately depress the tongue-tip to where the Cheerio was and hold for 1 second (1 unit).
   **Note:** Monitor to ensure the jaw is stable.
2. Criteria for Success: Repeat the unit described in #1, 50 times.
   Goals:

   1. Develop jaw-tongue dissociation
   2. Teach placement for dissociated tongue-tip elevation and depression as a component of mobility and agility during co-articulation

   Target Phonemes:

   / t, d, n, l, s, z, ʃ(sh), ʧ(ch), ʤ(j) / in conjunction with all vowels

## Step #3

1. If the target phoneme is / s / or / z /, proceed to Step #4. If the target phonemes are / t, d, n, l /, follow the direction for Step #3.
2. At this point, you are ready to introduce the standard production of:
   / t, d, n, l / in isolation.
   **Note:** Remember that prior to introducing this Step, you will have had to work on auditory awareness and auditory discrimination for your target phoneme.
3. Practice the target phonemes / t, d, n, or l / in isolation 50 times or until mastered.
4. Criteria for Success: Practice the target phoneme / t, d, n, or l / with the low jaw vowel "ah," 10 times, in each of the following nonsense syllables to ensure the tongue-tip elevates for the target phoneme and releases for the vowel. You will also be working on establishing a new **muscle memory,** the motor planning for lingual alveolar speech sounds.

   a. ta (10 times)    - at (10 times)    - ata (10 times)

   b. da (10 times)    - ad (10 times)    - ada (10 times)

186

c. na (10 times)  - an (10 times)  - ana (10 times)

d. la (10 times)  - al (10 times)  - ala (10 times)

5. Choose any traditional articulation therapy approach you feel comfortable with to work on carryover during and after this activity.

Goals:

1. Develop jaw-tongue dissociation

2. Teach placement for dissociated tongue-tip elevation and depression as a component of mobility and agility during co-articulation in conjunction with vowels.

Target Phonemes: / t, d, n, l /

Step #4

1. It is important to determine where your client should physiologically be making the / s / or / z /, with tongue-tip elevation or depression.

**Note:** During the past fifteen years of my lecturing, I have been conducting an informal research project. I have asked everyone in my classes to say an / s / in isolation and to determine where the tongue-tip is during the production of this sound. I then asked for a show of hands. "How many of you make your / s / with the tongue-tip up? How many of you make the / s / with the tongue-tip down? How many of you make your / s / with the tongue-tip in the middle?" Consistently, I have found diversity within each group. I then ask, "How many of you have a speech problem involving / s / or / z /?" Everyone laughs. But what have we learned? There are a variety of ways to make these sounds and the correct placement for each client is based on his or her oral structures and functions. The critical component is not in the position of the tongue-tip, but rather in the tension within the tongue-tip. The back of the tongue must be retracted with side spread, and the tongue-tip must be tensed for the standard production of / s / and / z /.

2. Place a tongue depressor between the **central incisors**, extending from the front of the mouth, as pictured in (a ). The tip of the tongue depressor should rest on the surface of the lower central incisors at midline. Instruct the client to bite down using a **natural bite** posture. Hold that position for 5 seconds.

**Note:**

a. If the jaw slides or juts in any direction despite numerous attempts to establish alignment, return to jaw stability activities.

b. If the client has a pronounced overbite, place the tongue depressor on the side teeth, extending from the side of the mouth, as pictured below in ( b ).

187

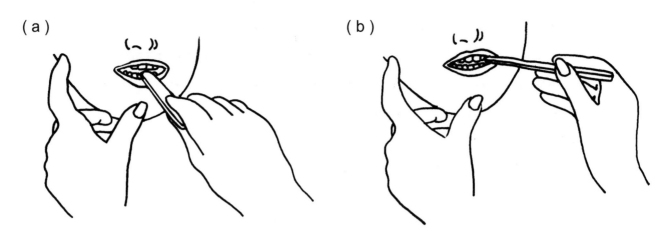

3. Criteria for Success: With the tongue depressor in place, instruct the client to elevate the tongue-tip to where the Cheerio was on the alveolar ridge and then to depress the tongue-tip to where the Cheerio was on the floor of the mouth, (1 unit) 5 times.

**Note:**
   a. If the jaw slides or juts in any direction despite numerous attempts to establish alignment, return to jaw stability activities.
   b. If the tongue depressor extends too far into the mouth, the tongue tip will not be able to make contact with the alveolar ridge.

Goals:
   1. Develop jaw-tongue dissociation
   2. Determine the optimal tongue-tip placement for / s / and / z /

Target Phonemes: / s, z /

Step #5

1. With the tongue depressor in place, instruct the client to say the sound of / ts / and then to "freeze" his/her tongue. Ask the client to "feel" where the tongue-tip is placed at the completion of the / ts /. Repeat this task until the client is able to identify the position of the tongue-tip consistently 5 times in one position.

2. Criteria for Success: With the tongue depressor in place, instruct the client to say the / ts /, extending the / s / for 2 to 3 seconds. Verbally reinforce where the client "feels" the tongue-tip, 10 times.

Goals:
   1. Develop jaw-tongue dissociation
   2. Determine the optimal tongue-tip placement for / s / and / z /

Target Phonemes: / s, z /

Step #6

1. With the tongue depressor in place, instruct the client to put his/her tongue-tip where it was for the 2 to 3 second production of / s /. Say / s / using this placement, 25 times in rapid succession.

2. Without the tongue depressor, instruct the client to put his/her tongue-tip where it was for the 2 to 3 second production of / s /. Say / s / using this placement, 25 times in rapid succession.

**Note:** Remember, prior to introducing the next level you will have had to work on auditory awareness and auditory discrimination for the target phoneme.

3. Practice the target phoneme / s / or / z / in isolation, 50 times.

4. Criteria for Success: Practice the target phoneme / s / or / z / with the low jaw vowel "ah," 10 times in each of the following nonsense syllables to ensure the tongue-tip elevates or depresses for the target phoneme and releases for the vowel. You will also be working on establishing a new **muscle memory** for the production of these sounds.

    a. sa (10 times)    - as (10 times)    - asa (10 times)

    b. za (10 times)    - az (10 times)    - aza (10 times)

5. Choose any traditional articulation therapy approach you feel comfortable with to work on **carryover** during and after this activity.

    Goals:

        1. Develop jaw-tongue dissociation

        2. Teach the optimal tongue-tip placement for the standard production of / s / or / z /

        3. Teach placement for dissociated tongue-tip elevation and depression as a component of mobility and agility during co-articulation

        4. Teach a new muscle memory pattern

    Target Phonemes

        / s / and / z / in isolation and in conjunction with the low jaw vowel "ah"

**Note:** Refer to *Oral Placement Therapy for / s / and / z /*, by Sara Rosenfeld-Johnson, SLP. In this program you will learn how to perform an evaluation with a client who evidences an inter-dental or a lateral "lisp," write a complete "Oral Placement/Movement for Feeding and Speech Evaluation," as well as create and write a "Program Plan" to address your client's specific needs. Once the process has been completed you will use the 20 Lesson Plans with associated Homework Sheets and Speech Practice Sheets to assist you in correcting your client's inter-dental or lateral productions.

# BACK OF TONGUE SIDE SPREAD - Summary
## Establishing Stability for Co-articulation

Standard co-articulation is based on the ability to stabilize the back of the tongue on the sides of the hard palate. This stabilizing posture will allow the remainder of the tongue to move independently in controlled dissociated patterns. The following activities, described earlier, should also be used to address the goal of back tongue side spread for stability and for the placement of the target phonemes: / i (ee), I (ih), ɛ (eh), ʃ(sh), tʃ(ch), ʤ(j), r, vocalic r /.

1. **Straw Drinking Hierarchy:** Refer to the complete explanation of the technique, described in this book. Clients who are only working on back of tongue side spread will begin this technique with Straw #4.

   **Note:** Refer to the video, *Straws as Therapy Tools*, for a complete visual demonstration of this technique for yourself, parents, teachers, etc.

2. **Horn Blowing Hierarchy:** Refer to the complete explanation of the technique, described in this book. Clients who are only working on back of tongue side spread will begin this technique with Horn #9.

   **Note:** Refer to the video, *Horns as Therapy Tools*, for a complete visual demonstration of this technique for yourself, parents, teachers, etc.

3. **Bubble Blowing Hierarchy:** Refer to the complete explanation of the technique, described in this book. Clients who are only working on back of tongue side spread, will begin this technique with Step #6.

   **Note:** Refer to the video, *Bubbles as Therapy Tools,* for a complete visual demonstration of this technique for yourself, parents, teachers, etc.

# "EE" Tongue Placement Production Criteria for / ʃ (sh), ʧ(ch), ʤ(j)/

One therapy technique which many of us have tried in the past uses the standard production of "ee" as a starting point to teach the vocalic / r /. Both the "ee" and the vocalic / r / have back of tongue side spread in common. In the production of "ee," we are able to use jaw elevation to assist in establishing and maintaining the tongue placement, whereas in the production of the vocalic / r / the jaw is not able to help. The difference, therefore, is jaw-tongue dissociation. If your client has jaw-tongue dissociation, the "ee" technique will work. If your client does not have jaw-tongue dissociation, the "ee" technique will not be effective.

This activity is designed to teach awareness, placement, mobility and muscle memory for back of tongue side spread. At the conclusion of this activity, you will have taught the standard tongue placement for the production of: / ʃ(sh), ʧ(ch), ʤ(j)/

The specific oral placement and movement goals are listed after each Step.

Suggestions:

1. You will need to 5 to 25 empty, clean junior baby food jars and 5 to 25 small toys that can fit , one each, inside the jars to implement this activity.
2. Homework: Establish during the session where the client fails on the hierarchy. Practice that Step at the highest level of successful repetitions for at least one week before moving on to the next level or Step.

Step #1

1. If the client is able to say "ee" without additional motivation, progress to Step #2.
2. Place a single item (e.g., Fisher-Price Little People) in an empty, clean junior baby food jar. Make sure the lid is tightened only slightly on the jar.
3. Use 5 jars with a single motivator inside each jar.
4. Criteria for Success: Instruct the client to say "ee" as he/she removes the lid from each of the 5 jars. Empty the contents of each jar into a basket to be used later during the language segment of your therapy session.

    **Note:** You may want to pretend the jars are difficult to open and you have to work hard to release the lid. The charade will help the less cooperative client to feel success and to associate the "ee" with the task.

    Goals:
    1. Teach placement for back of tongue side spread
    2. Develop jaw-tongue dissociation

<u>Target Phonemes:</u>  / i (ee), I (ih),  ɛ (eh), ʃ(sh), tʃ(ch), ʤ(j), r, vocalic r /

<u>Step #2</u>

1.  Use the motivator suggested in Step #1 if necessary.

2.  <u>Criteria for Success:</u>  Instruct the client to say "ee" 25 times.

    <u>Goals:</u>

    1.  Teach placement for back of tongue side spread

    2.  Develop jaw-tongue dissociation


<u>Target Phonemes:</u>  / i (ee), I (ih),  ɛ (eh), ʃ(sh), tʃ(ch), ʤ(j), r, vocalic r /


<u>Step #3</u>

1.  As the client says "ee," ask him/her to describe what he/she is feeling in the mouth. "Do you feel how the sides of your tongue in the back are touching the top of your palate or the upper back molars?"

2.  Criteria for Success:  Show Picture #1, below, of the hard palate and upper teeth. Ask the client to show you where on the picture his/her tongue is touching the hard palate or the upper back molar ridges.  If the placement is correct, as demonstrated in Picture #2, progress to Step #6.  If not, progress to Step #4.

Picture #1

Picture #2

<u>Goals:</u>

1.  Teach placement for back of tongue side spread

2.  Develop jaw-tongue dissociation

3.  Teach awareness of the "feel" of back of the tongue side spread, stabilizing on the back of the palate and/or on the upper back molar ridges, to teach placement for the standard production of:  / ʃ(sh), tʃ(ch), ʤ(j), r, vocalic r /


<u>Target Phonemes:</u>  / i (ee), I (ih),  ɛ (eh), ʃ(sh), tʃ(ch), ʤ(j), r, vocalic r /

## Step #4

1. At this point, it will be necessary to increase the client's awareness of where the tongue is stabilizing to teach placement for the standard production of: / ʃ(sh), tʃ(ch), dʒ(j), r, vocalic r /

2. Instruct the client to open his/her mouth wide. Use a Q-tip to touch the sides of the back of the tongue along the lateral margins. Confirm that your client can feel where you are touching.

3. Instruct the client to say "ee." Ask what he/she is feeling in the mouth. "Do you feel how the sides of your tongue in the back are touching the top of your palate or your upper back molars?"

4. <u>Criteria for Success:</u> Show Picture #1, on the previous page, of the hard palate and upper teeth. Ask the client to show you where on the picture his/her tongue is touching the hard palate and/or upper back upper teeth. If the placement is correct, as demonstrated in Picture #2, progress to Step #6. If not, progress to Step #5.

   <u>Goals:</u>

   1. Teach placement for back of tongue side spread

   2. Develop jaw-tongue dissociation

   3. Teach awareness of the "feel" of back of the tongue side spread, stabilizing on the back of the palate and/or on the back molar ridges, to teach placement for the standard production of: / ʃ(sh), tʃ(ch), dʒ(j), r, vocalic r /


   <u>Target Phonemes:</u> / i (ee), I (ih), ε (eh), ʃ(sh), tʃ(ch), dʒ(j), r, vocalic r /


## Step #5

1. Instruct the client to open his/her mouth wide. Use a Q-tip dipped in a highly-flavored liquid or extract (i.e., lemon, mint) to touch the lateral margins at the back of the tongue. Confirm that your client can feel where you are touching.

2. Instruct the client to say "ee." Ask what he/she is feeling in the mouth. "Do you feel how the sides of the back of your tongue are touching the top of your palate or the upper back teeth?"

3. Criteria for Success: Show Picture #1 of the hard palate and upper teeth. Ask the client to show you where on the picture his/her tongue is touching the hard palate and/or back upper molar ridge, to confirm the placement is correct, as demonstrated in Picture #2. If the placement is correct, progress to Step #6.

Goals:

1. Teach placement for back of tongue side spread
2. Develop jaw-tongue dissociation
3. Teach awareness of the "feel" of back of the tongue side spread, stabilizing on the back of the palate and/or on the back molar ridges, to teach placement for the standard production of:  / ʃ(sh), ʧ(ch), ʤ(j), r, vocalic r /

Target Phonemes:  / i (ee), I (ih),  ɛ (eh), ʃ(sh), ʧ(ch), ʤ(j), r, vocalic r /


## Step #6

1. Instruct the client to say "ee."  Confirm that he/she is feeling the correct placement. Have the client make a "funny face" to ensure the tongue moves away from the palate.

   **Note:** With older clients or cognitively intact clients, you may choose to just tell them to move the tongue away from the palate.

2. Criteria for Success:  Have the client repeat #1, 50 times.  Intermittently remind the client to feel the correct tongue placement.

   Goals:

   1. Teach placement for back of tongue side spread
   2. Develop jaw-tongue dissociation
   3. Teach awareness of the "feel" of back of the tongue side spread, stabilizing on the back of the palate and/or on the back molar ridges, to teach placement for the standard production of:  / ʃ(sh), ʧ(ch), ʤ(j), r, vocalic r /

   Target Phonemes:  / i (ee), I (ih),  ɛ (eh), ʃ(sh), ʧ(ch), ʤ(j), r, vocalic r  /


## Step #7

1. Instruct the client to achieve the "ee" placement and to freeze the tongue and the jaw in that posture.
2. Criteria for Success:  While maintaining this frozen posture, instruct the client to move only his/her lips to say the sound of your target phoneme.  Your choices will be to target / ʃ(sh), ʧ(ch), ʤ(j), r / or the vocalic / r /.  Visually demonstrate the production placement of this phoneme 5 times.  If the production is standard, progress to Step #8.

194

**Note:**

    a. If you have targeted the vocalic / r / and the placement production of that phoneme is not correct, progress to the activity entitled, "Dinosaur for / r /."

    b. If you have targeted / ʃ(sh), tʃ(ch), dʒ(j) / and the tongue placement is correct but there is insufficient lip rounding/protrusion, return to "Lip Activities."

    c. If you have targeted / tʃ(ch) / or / dʒ(j) / and the client is substituting / ʃ(sh) / for these targeted phonemes, return to the activity, "Cheerio for Tongue-Tip Elevation."

    d. If you have targeted / ʃ(sh), tʃ(ch), dʒ(j) / and the tongue placement of these phonemes is lateralized, return to "Tongue Activities" to work on tongue grading and dissociation.

  Goals:

    1. Teach placement for back of tongue side spread

    2. Develop jaw-tongue dissociation

    3. Teach awareness of the "feel" of back of the tongue side  spread, stabilizing on the back of the palate and/or on the back molar ridges, to teach placement for the standard production of:  / ʃ(sh), tʃ(ch), dʒ(j), r, vocalic r /

Target Phonemes:  / ʃ(sh), tʃ(ch), dʒ(j), r, vocalic r /


Step #8

1. Repeat the standard production of your target phoneme / ʃ(sh), tʃ(ch), dʒ(j), r, vocalic r /, 50 times in the frozen posture.

2. Instruct the client to say the target phoneme  / ʃ(sh), tʃ(ch), dʒ(j), r, vocalic r /, 1 time in the frozen posture.  Have the client make a "funny face" to ensure the tongue moves away from the palate.

  **Note:** With older clients or cognitively intact clients, you may choose to just tell them to move the tongue away from the palate.

3. Have the client repeat 2. in this step 50 times.  Intermittently, remind the client to "feel" the correct tongue placement.

4. Criteria for Success:  Repeat the standard production of your target phoneme 50 times in isolation before progressing on to the word level.

5. Choose any traditional articulation therapy program you feel comfortable with to work on carry-over during or after this activity.

195

Goals:

1. Teach placement for back of tongue side spread

2. Develop jaw-tongue dissociation

3. Teach awareness of the "feel" of back of the tongue side spread, stabilizing on the back of the palate and/or on the back molar ridges, to teach placement for the standard production of:  / ʃ(sh), tʃ(ch), dʒ(j), r, vocalic r /

Target Phonemes:  / ʃ(sh), tʃ(ch), dʒ(j), r, vocalic r /

# DINOSAUR FOR / r / Production Criteria for /r/ and the vocalic / r /

This activity is designed to teach awareness, placement, mobility and muscle memory in the three muscle groups which make up the standard production of the vocalic / r /: jaw, lips and tongue. At the conclusion of this activity you will introduce the standard production of the vocalic / r /. Before introducing this technique it will be important to understand the standard articulator placement and movements for the vocalic / r / and to then determine which of these muscle movements your client is doing incorrectly. Because the jaw, lips and tongue placement are involved in the production, deficits in one, two or all three muscle functions will result in a distortion of the clarity of the speech sound.

1. Jaw: Jaw-tongue dissociation is critical for the co-articulated movement which is a component of the vocalic / r /. Rest your flat palm under your jaw as you say a standard vocalic / r / aloud. "Feel" your jaw position. What you are feeling is a High to Medium Jaw Height. Now say the vocalic / r / as your client would say it. What happened to your jaw? If it dropped, you have identified that at least one of your client's goals will be to achieve a higher jaw position during the production of the vocalic / r /.

2. Lips: Jaw-lip dissociation is critical for the standard production of the vocalic / r /. Place the ball of your pointer finger under your lower lip at midline as you say a standard vocalic / r / aloud. "Feel" your lip position. What you are feeling is slight tension in the muscles under the lower lip. Now say the vocalic / r / as your client would say it. What happens to your lips? If your lips round, you have identified that your client is using the orbicularis-oris instead of the mentalis muscle system to make the vocalic / r /. At least one of your goals will be to create awareness, placement, mobility and muscle memory in the mentalis muscle system.

3. Tongue: Jaw-lip-tongue dissociation is critical for the standard production of the vocalic / r /. With many of our clients, the jaw is being used to help the tongue maintain placement. Begin by saying a standard vocalic / r / aloud. "Feel" your tongue placement. There are two possibilities here for **Target Placement**:

    a. Back of tongue side spread: This is the most common placement and is characterized by the back of the lateral margins of the tongue making contact with the back of the palate. In some cases, the sides of the tongue spread over to the molar ridges, as pictured below.

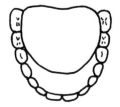

b. <u>Backing up placement</u>: This placement is less common, but also standard. This placement results in a back of tongue side spread which does not make contact with the palate or molar ridges during the isolated production of the vocalic / r /, but does do so at the conversational speech level.

Now say the vocalic / r / as your client would say it. What happens to your tongue? If it drops, loses its spread, or tightens into a retracted ball, at least one of your goals will be to teach a back of tongue side spread which does not rely on the jaw to maintain its position.

Each of the placement deficits identified in "b" has been addressed in previous activities. The group of activities entitled, "Dinosaur for / r /," will be the last technique you will attempt for clients with a vocalic / r / distortion. It is a technique which incorporates all of the isolated movements needed to produce the vocalic / r / into one controlled movement. Therefore, prior to introducing "Dinosaur for / r /," return to the appropriate activities listed below to determine if the client has achieved the necessary placement criteria to begin "Dinosaur for / r /."

1. Jaw Stability/Grading Exercises must be completed before introducing "Dinosaur for / r /."
   a. Bite Block (Jaw Heights #2 through #7)
   b. Twin Bite Blocks for Symmetrical Jaw Stability (Jaw Heights #2 through #7)
   c. Tongue Depressor for Jaw Stability (Jaw Heights #2 through #7)
2. The activity that will increase awareness, placement, mobility and muscle memory in the mentalis muscle system is entitled, "Tongue Depressor for Lip Closure." It must be completed before introducing "Dinosaur for / r /."
3. The activities that will increase awareness, placement, mobility and muscle memory for proper tongue placement which must be completed before introducing "Dinosaur for / r /" are:
   a. "Horn Blowing Hierarchy"
   b. "Straw Drinking Hierarchy"
   c. "EE"

Once the client has achieved the Criteria for Success in each of the activities listed above, you are ready to introduce "Dinosaur for / r /."

The specific oral placement and movement goals are listed after each Step.

<u>Suggestions:</u>

1. It is important to remember that many of these clients have been receiving traditional speech therapy for a number of years. The reason that traditional therapy has not worked with these clients is that they have a placement and movement disorder. Therefore, before introducing this technique, you should spend some time explaining

the following to your client. It is not the fault of the client that he/she has been having so much trouble learning to say the targeted speech sound. It is not the fault of the speech therapist either. This way of looking at the placement and movement of muscles for the production of / r / is new. At the conclusion of this conversation, you may tell the client not to practice saying any / r / words as we will be practicing placement and movements to help you to say this sound correctly.

**Note:** Traditional speech therapy has been highly successful for clients with speech sound phonological disorders and/or Auditory Awareness/Discrimination Disorders. Traditional speech therapy has not been effective for clients who cannot produce the sound correctly with only auditory and verbal cuing.

2. You will need a tongue depressor with 16 pennies attached to it to implement this activity. Refer to the activity entitled, "Tongue Depressor for Lip Closure" for directions on how to make this therapy tool.

3. Homework: Establish during the session where the client fails on the hierarchy. Practice that Step at the highest level of successful repetitions for at least one week before moving on to the next level or Step.


Step #1

1. Instruct the client to produce an "ee" sound in isolation. Verify that he/she can "feel" the back of the tongue side spread stabilizing on the back of the palate.

   **Note:** If the client cannot "feel" this placement, refer to the activity entitled, "EE."

2. Have the client repeat the production of "ee" using a "robot voice" (i.e., glottal fry). Ask, "Where is the back of your tongue when you are saying this sound?" Make sure the response is that it is touching the location identified in the picture on page 197 (**Target Placement**).

   **Note:** You will not be using this component of the technique long enough to develop a voice disorder. The purpose of teaching the "ee" with a glottal fry is to establish the placement of the sound in the oral cavity. You should try this technique yourself before using it with a client. Begin by saying a standard vocalic / r / a loud. "Feel" the placement of the sound in your mouth. What you are feeling is the sound being made back and high in the mouth. Now say the vocalic / r / as your client would say it. What happens to the placement of the sound? It moves forward.

199

3. <u>Criteria for Success:</u> Have the client repeat the "ee," using the "robot voice," 25 times. Continue to remind the client to feel the tongue placement each time

<u>Goals:</u>

1. "Feel" back of tongue side spread stabilizing on the back of the hard palate and/or upper back molars

2. Associate the placement of "ee" in "robot voice" with high, back placement in the mouth

<u>Target Phoneme:</u> vocalic / r /


## <u>Step #2</u>

1. Instruct the client to say "ee" in the "robot voice" and then to immediately say "eh" in the "robot voice," (1 unit), without moving the tongue away from the point of stability (i.e., **target placement** on the hard palate/molars).

**<u>Note:</u>** "Eh" is used in this activity to teach jaw-tongue dissociation. In the production of "ee," the jaw is in a High position, whereas in the production of "eh," the jaw drops to a Medium Jaw Height. Without jaw-tongue dissociation, the tongue could not maintain the target placement during the production of "eh."

2. <u>Criteria for Success:</u> Repeat 1. (1 unit) 25 times. Continue to remind the client to feel the targeted tongue placement, throughout this activity.

<u>Goals:</u>

1. Associate back of tongue side spread stabilizing on the back of the hard palate and/or upper back molars with the production of "eh"

2. Teach jaw-tongue dissociation

<u>Target Phoneme:</u> vocalic / r /


## <u>Step #3</u>

1. Instruct the client to establish the tongue placement for "ee" silently, then without moving the tongue off of the targeted position to say "eh" using the "robot voice" (1 unit), 1 time.

2. <u>Criteria for Success:</u> Repeat 1. (1 unit) 25 times. Continue to remind the client to feel the targeted tongue placement, throughout this activity.

<u>Goals:</u>

1. Associate back of tongue side spread stabilizing on the back of the hard palate and/or upper back molars with the production of "eh"

2. Teach jaw-tongue dissociation

<u>Target Phoneme:</u> vocalic / r /

Step #4

1. Place a tongue depressor with 8 pennies affixed to each end between the client's closed lips (as practiced in the activity entitled "Tongue Depressor for Lip Closure"). Hold this position for 5 seconds. Make the client aware of the tension in the muscle system below his/her lower lip.

2. Instruct the client to "freeze" his/her lips in this position as you remove the tongue depressor. When the tongue depressor has been removed, the existing lip placement can now be known as the "Duckbill Dinosaur Lip Position."

3. Practice establishing the "Duckbill Dinosaur Lip Position" without the tongue depressor. Once the position is achieved, use a mirror to reinforce the placement.

   **Note:**

   a. For some clients, you may have to alternate between using the tongue depressor and not using the tongue depressor as a transition phase.

   b. When working with a client with motor planning difficulties including apraxia or dyspraxia, you should alternate between using the tongue depressor and not using the tongue depressor to assist in motor planning.

4. Criteria for Success:    Practice the "Duckbill Dinosaur Lip Position," 25 times, without using the tongue depressor.

   Goals:

   1. Teach jaw-lip dissociation
   2. Teach the "Duckbill Dinosaur Lip Position"

   Target Phoneme: vocalic / r /


Step #5

1. In this Step you will combine the standard jaw, lip and tongue positions for the placement of the vocalic / r / by combining Step #3 and Step #4 without saying the targeted sound.

2. Instruct the client to say the "eh" using the "robot voice" with the back of the tongue in the target position and then to immediately place his/her lips in the Duckbill Dinosaur Lip Position without moving the jaw or tongue  (1 unit).

   **Note:** It is important the client stops vocalizing as he/she makes the transition to the Duckbill Dinosaur Lip Position.

3. Criteria for Success: Repeat 2. (1 unit), 25 times. Continue to remind the client not to move the jaw or tongue placement throughout this activity.

201

Goals:
  1. Teach jaw-lip-tongue dissociation
  2. Teach standard placement and movement of jaw, lips and tongue to teach standard production of the vocalic / r /

Target Phoneme: vocalic / r /


Step #6

  1. Instruct the client to say the "eh" using the "robot voice" with the back of the tongue in the targeted placement and then to continue to vocalize, using the "robot voice," as he/she places the lips in the Duckbill Dinosaur Lip Position (1 unit).

  **Note:** Monitor to ensure the client is not moving the jaw or tongue throughout this activity.

  2. Criteria for Success: Repeat 1. (1 unit), 25 times. Continue to remind the client not to move the tongue or jaw throughout this activity.

  Goals:
    1. Teach jaw-lip-tongue dissociation
    2. Teach standard placement and movement of jaw, lips and tongue to teach standard production of the vocalic / r /

  Target Phoneme: vocalic / r /


Step #7

  1. Instruct the client:
    a. Say the "eh" using the "robot voice" with the back of the tongue in the targeted position and then
    b. Inhale and continue to vocalize in a "sigh," without using the "robot voice," as you place your lips in the Duckbill Dinosaur Lip Position, (1 unit).

  **Note:** Monitor to ensure the client is not moving the jaw or tongue throughout this activity.

  2. Criteria for Success: Repeat 1. (1 unit), 25 times. Continue to remind the client not to move the tongue or jaw throughout this activity.

  Goals:
    1. Teach jaw-lip-tongue dissociation
    2. Teach standard placement and movement of jaw, lips and tongue to teach standard production of the vocalic / r /

  Target Phoneme: vocalic / r /

Step #8

1. Instruct the client:

   a. "Think" the "eh," as you place your tongue and jaw in the target position and then

   b. Immediately place your lips in the Duckbill Dinosaur Lip Position.

   c. While maintaining this standard placement of jaw, lips and tongue, say the vocalic / r / 1 time.

2. If the production is standard, progress to 4. If it is not produced in the standard manner, progress to 3.

3. Repeat the instructions in 1. reminding the client to inhibit all movement in the jaw, lips and tongue once the standard placement is established.

4. Criteria for Success: Repeat the technique described in 1. (1 unit), using the standard production of the vocalic / r /, 25 times.

   Goals:

   1. Teach jaw-lip-tongue dissociation

   2. Teach standard placement and movement of jaw, lips and tongue to teach standard production of the vocalic / r /

   Target Phoneme: vocalic / r /

Step #9

1. At this point, you are ready to continue the standard production of the vocalic / r / in isolation.

   **Note:** Remember that prior to introducing this Step, you will have had to work on a auditory awareness and auditory discrimination for your target phoneme.

2. Instruct the client to put his/her jaw, lips and tongue in the standard placement as described in Step #8 and to say the sound of the vocalic / r /.

3. Criteria for Success: Repeat the standard production of your target phoneme 50 times or until mastered, before progressing to the word level.

4. Choose any traditional therapy approach that you feel comfortable with to work on carryover.

   Goals:

   1. Teach jaw-lip-tongue dissociation

   2. Teach standard placement and movement of jaw, lips and tongue to teach standard production of the vocalic / r /

   Target Phoneme: vocalic / r /

# SAMPLE PROGRAM PLAN COMPONENTS

Initial Program Plans - Each technique/activity is introduced in the initial therapy session. Once the highest level before failure has been identified in the therapy session, that level is recorded on the "TalkTools® Oral Placement Homework Chart" and sent home for daily practice. This form can be found in the DVD *Forms for Oral-Motor Assesment and Treatment*, by Sara Rosenfeld-Johnson, SLP. Each subsequent weekly therapy session is designed to identify gains, increase the number of repetitions or to introduce new techniques as skills are mastered.

**Note:** The following Program Plan lists only the elements of a Program Plan. It does not include descriptions of each element as would be included in a real Program Plan. When I write a real Program Plan I include specific information based on the results of a Complete Oral Placement for Speech and Feeding Assessment. The Program Plan is being included in this book to assist you in understanding how a therapy session is organized. For further information on how to diagnose and treat Oral Placement and Movement deficits, refer to the videos titled: *Level 2: Diagnosis and Program Planning for Clients with Oral-Motor Based Articulation Disorders,* by Sara Rosenfeld-Johnson, SLP, (TalkTools® 2003); *Level 2: Oral-Motor Therapy: Assessment and Program Plan Development* by Renee Roy Hill, SLP (TalkTools® 2009)

1.  Sensory:
    a.  Therapeutic Seating
    b.  Work with hands down or at midline
    c.  Toothette with Vibration - across midline
    d.  Inhibit all compensatory postures

2.  Feeding:
    a.  Liquids: Straw Drinking for Thin Liquids: Straw #1 - cut to ¾" above lip block
    b.  Purees: Pointed Spoon Slurp - 6 slurps at the beginning of each meal then finish the rest of the puree in the habitual pattern to ensure nutritional intake
    c.  Solids: Small Plate - Large Plate - 2 cubes per side per meal on back molars then finish the rest of the solids in the habitual manner to ensure nutritional intake

3.  Oral Placement Activities:
    a.  Bubble Blowing Hierarchy - Level 2 - 3 breaths, 2 times
    b.  Horn Blowing Hierarchy - Horn #1 - 4 blows, 2 times

c. Jaw Grading Bite Blocks - #2 Bite Block - Exercise A - 2 seconds per side, 10 times

d. Slow Feed - 2 bites per side, 10 times

4. Speech: Always continue to work on developing receptive and expressive language skills. Vocabulary beginning with /m b, or p/ should be targeted as this child can produce these phonemes in the standard manner both acoustically and at the motor level using standard placement. The above described Program Plan addresses the placement and movement components of speech production. As adequate mobility and endurance are achieved for the oral articulators addressed in this Program Plan, direct work on production of speech sounds will be enhanced.

## Recommendations:

1. The above prescribed Program Plan should be implemented a minimum of three times per week for 15-20 minutes. Since the tasks described above will only be changed one time per week, this client should be seen at least one time per week by a trained SLP. The other two practice sessions can be implemented by the parent, teacher, aide, etc.

2. This Program Plan is being recommended to supplement the existing speech and language intervention, not to replace it.

# GLOSSARY

**Adding Weight:** Applying pressure to a given muscle or muscle group to the degree that it increases awareness but does not move the muscle.

**Articulation:** In speech, a series of overlapping movements which places varying degrees of obstruction in the path of the outgoing air stream and simultaneously involves accuracy in placement of the articulators, timing, direction of movements, force extended, speed of response. The movements include dissociation and grading in the following muscle groups: abdomen, larynx, velum, jaw, lips, tongue.

**Assimilation Nasality:** Hypernasality occurring only on those sounds which immediately precede (regressive assimilation) the nasal consonants / m /, / n /, / ng /.

**Assisted Jaw Stability:** A technique used to help a weak jaw to remain stable so that other oral muscles can improve their functional levels. Example: Supporting the client's jaw with the palm of your hand.

**Assisted Jaw Elevation:** A technique used to reposition the weak jaw to assist in lip closure exercises. Example: Closing the jaw, without forcing it, to give the client the feel of a High Jaw Position.

**Assisted Lip Closure:** A technique used to reposition the lips to enable the client to perform a lip closure exercise. Example: Holding the lips together to teach the lip approximation position for blowing a flat-mouthed horn.

**Assisted Lip Rounding:** A technique used to reposition the lips to enable the client to perform a lip rounding exercise. Example: Holding the sides of the lips, while using your fingers to push the lips slightly towards midline to teach the lip rounding/protrusion position for drinking from a straw.

**Asymmetry:** Unequal balance of structure, skill levels or movement. Unequal movement in corresponding extremities or muscle groups on opposites of the body.

**Auditorially Based Standard Phoneme Production:** A situation where the phoneme sounds to be normal or standard based on the listener's hearing of that phoneme.

**Auditory Awareness:** A traditional speech therapy technique which utilizes the auditory feedback system to create and maintain standard speech sound clarity.

**Bite Block:** Any firm texture that inhibits the mobility of the jaw when bitten.

**Bolus:** Any food mass within the oral cavity.

**Carry-over:** The ability to transition a movement, skill or speech sound into habit.

**Central Incisors:** The two upper and two lower teeth at mouth midline.

**Co-articulation:** Articulatory movements for one phone which are carried over into the previous or subsequent phones but which do not affect the primary place of articulation. The transition from one phoneme to another in connected speech.

**Compensatory Pattern:** Any pattern that is used to substitute for a movement that is not physiologically possible.

**Criteria for Success:** The skill that must be completed successfully so that the client can progress to the next highest level of function.

**Dietary Issues:** Food intake limitations secondary to function, allergic reaction, religious restrictions or family preferences.

**Dissociation:** The separation of movement based on strength/stability in one or more muscle groups.

**Duration:** The length of time it takes to complete a movement or an action.

**Eight Levels of Tongue Grading:** The eight segmented areas of the tongue that must have strength/ stability to allow for dissociation of lingual movements for normal feeding skill development, oral placement activity completion and standard speech clarity.

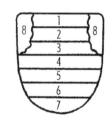

**Elongation:** Increasing the length of a muscle or group of muscles.

**Exhalation:** The action of releasing air from the lungs as a component of breathing or through controlled abdominal muscle grading during speech sound production.

**Existing Bubble:** After blowing a bubble from a bubble wand, that bubble is then balanced on the same wand.

**Eye Level:** A position for working with a client that facilitates a 90 degree angle in the chin, thereby, inhibiting the client from having to look up or to look down to see the instructor.

**Facial Cueing:** A tactile teaching technique which touches or manipulates the oral articulators as a means of assisting in speech sound production.

**Favorite Liquid:** At the start of therapy, ask the client or the client's parent to list those liquids that are especially enjoyed by the client. Also, ask for those liquids which the client prefers, but rarely has, because of limited nutritional value. These liquids will eventually become motivators for the more difficult oral placement activities.

**Fine Motor:** Use of the small muscles of the hand, as well as the coordination of the eyes and hand together to manipulate objects.

**Fixing:** An abnormal posture used to compensate for reduced stability which inhibits mobility.

**Fluctuating Nasality:** An inability to consistently control the nasal airflow associated with speech sound production.

**Fluctuating Sensitivity:** Sensitivity which changes over time.

**Grading:** The controlled segmentation of movement based upon strength, stability and dissociation. The ability to control movement at any point through the range of movement. Gross Motor: Quality, strength and flexibility of active large muscle movement including coordination, balance and locomotion.

**Habit:** An act or movement that has become automatic.

**High Jaw Fixed Posture:** An abnormal compensatory pattern characterized by immobility in the jaw at Jaw Height #1, #2 or #3, secondary to jaw weakness and insufficient jaw grading.

**High Jaw Posture:** One of the three levels of controlled jaw grading. Stability at Jaw Height #1, #2 and #3 (High Jaw Posture) will translate into normal jaw functioning at these jaw heights for feeding, oral placement activities and for speech sound production. (Refer to the diagram under "Jaw Height Hierarchy" on the next page.)

**Highly Flavored Licorice:** A therapy product that comes in five flavors: grape, cinnamon, sour apple, lemon and raspberry. When left outside of the package for two to three days, they will harden without becoming brittle. They can then be used as Bite Blocks or to teach a munch pattern for chewing. When fresh, they can be used for a taste bud analysis and to teach lateralization across midline.

**Hypernasality:** Excessive nasal airflow during speech sound production, secondary to structural or functional deficits in the velopharyngeal mechanism.

**Hypersensitivity:** An overreaction to sensory input.

**Hyponasality:** Insufficient nasal airflow during the production of standard nasalized speech sounds / m, n, ng /.

**Hypo-sensitivity:** An underreaction to sensory input.

**Ice Finger:** A therapy tool which is made by filling the fingers of a clean latex glove with water 3/4 of the way up. The glove is then hung up in a freezer until it is solid. When needed, the gloved ice finger is cut. The remaining end of that latex glove finger that is not filled with ice is tied in a knot to prevent dripping as the ice melts. This pointed therapy tool can now be used for thermal sensory work.

209

**Independent Self-Feeding:** A situation where the individual is placing the food in his or her mouth without assistance.

**Inhalation:** The action of drawing air into the lungs for breathing or to support controlled airflow for speech sound production.

**Isometric Pull:** Adding a forward pull that is just strong enough to keep the muscle from losing its hold on an object.

**Jaw Height Hierarchy:** The eight graded levels that translate into controlled elevation and depression movements of the jaw that are prerequisites for achieving normal feeding skill development, oral placement activity completion and standard speech clarity.

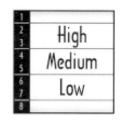

**Jaw Jut:** A one directional abnormal movement of the jaw which can be observed to the right, to the left or to the front. This type of jaw instability is generally secondary to asymmetrical jaw strength.

**Jaw Slide:** An abnormal jaw movement which is fluid, thereby, multi-directional. This type of jaw instability is generally secondary to symmetrical jaw weakness.

**Jaw-Lip Dissociation:** The ability to move the jaw and lips independently of each other during function.

**Jaw-Lip-Tongue Dissociation:** The ability to move the jaw, lips and tongue independently of each other during function. This level of dissociation is a prerequisite for the development of normal feeding skills and standard, co-articulated speech clarity.

**Kinesthetic Feedback:** A sense mediated by end organs located in muscles, tendons, and joints which is stimulated by bodily movement and tensions. In speech, the awareness of the location of the articulators during the production of phonemes.

**Laffy Taffy:** A therapy product that comes in a variety of flavors. When refrigerated, it will harden. It can then be used as a Bite Block or to teach a munch pattern for chewing.

**Lip Block:** Any item that inhibits the lips from moving further onto the straw. The lip block is designed to inhibit lingual suckling and biting.

**Low Jaw Fixed Posture:** An abnormal compensatory pattern characterized by immobility in the jaw at Jaw Height #6, #7 or #8, secondary to jaw weakness and insufficient jaw grading.

**Low Jaw Posture:** One of the three levels of controlled jaw grading. Stability at Jaw Height #6, #7 and #8 (Low Jaw Posture) will translate into normal jaw functioning at these jaw heights for feeding and for speech sound production. (Refer to the diagram under "Jaw Height Hierarchy" above.)

**Medium Jaw Fixed Posture:** A compensatory pattern characterized by immobility in the jaw at Jaw Height #4 or #5, secondary to jaw weakness and insufficient jaw grading.

**Medium Jaw Posture:** One of the three levels of controlled jaw grading. Stability at Jaw Height #4 and #5 (Medium Jaw Posture) will translate into normal jaw functioning at these jaw heights for feeding and for speech sound production. (Refer to the diagram under "Jaw Height Hierarchy" on the previous page.)

**Midline:** An imaginary line that divides a structure or muscle group in half. The median plane of the body.

**Mixed Sensitivity:** A combination of hypersensitivity, hyposensitivity and/or normal sensitivity.

**Motor Planning:** The ability to sequence movements that are necessary to perform a task. The ability of the brain to conceive, organize, and carry out a sequence of unfamiliar actions. This is also known as praxis.

**Munch Chew:** A chew that is characterized by an up and down movement.

**Muscle Memory:** The habit that makes a movement automatic.

**Nasal Airflow:** Air that is released through the nasal passage during breathing, oral exercise or during speech sound production.

**Natural Bite:** The optimal bite alignment that can be achieved with the existing jaw and dental structures.

**NDT (Neuro-Developmental Technique):** A field of study that teaches that development follows a hierarchy of movement based upon the establishment of skills at sequential levels within the body. A technique aimed at the inhibition of abnormal reflex activity and the facilitation of normal patterns.

**Normal Muscle Movement:** The standardized age appropriate skill levels in muscle control based upon strength, stability, dissociation and grading.

**Obligatory Mouth Breather:** The reliance upon inhalation and exhalation of air for breathing through the mouth, secondary to blockage or air passage restrictions in the nasal cavity.

**OPT Articulation Form:** A form used to transcribe the placement locations of phonemes used in standardized articulation tests. Available through TalkTools at: www.talktools.com

**Oral Airflow:** Air that is released through the oral cavity/mouth during breathing, oral exercise or during speech sound production.

**Oral Placement Therapy (OPT):** Speech therapy which utilizes a combination of: (1) auditory stimulation, (2) visual stimulation and (3) tactile stimulation to the mouth to improve speech clarity. This technique teaches only speech-like movements.

**Phonation:** Physiological process whereby the energy of moving air in the vocal tract is transformed into acoustic energy within the larynx. Production of voiced sound by means of vocal fold vibration.

**Phoneme:** A family of sounds that function in a language to signal a difference in meaning. Shortest arbitrary unit of sound in a given language that can be recognized as being distinct from other sounds in the language.

**Phonological Disorder:** Characterized by difficulty understanding the rules used for combining sounds to produce words which results in sound system errors.

**Placement:** The position of an articulator during function which is limited to an isolated movement, thereby, requiring minimal strength and endurance.

**Positive Reinforcement:** A behavior modification technique which rewards the client for task completion.

**Production:** The ability to work on the verbal component of a phoneme, saying the sound, based upon completion of the prerequisite skill levels of: (1) awareness, (2) placement, and (3) adequate strength/muscle memory.

**Program Plan:** The oral placement for feeding and speech therapy goals and techniques that are created for the client based upon diagnostic testing. Program Plans are divided into four areas which should be addressed simultaneously: (1) sensory system, (2) feeding, (3) OPT activities, and (4) speech.

**Resonation:** A quality imparted to voiced sounds by vibration in anatomical resonating chambers or cavities, such as the mouth or the nasal cavity.

**Respiration:** A single complete act of breathing which includes equal parts of inhalation and exhalation.

**Sensory Integration:** The organization of sensory information for use. The "use" may be a perception of the body or the world, or an adaptive response, or a learning process, or the development of some neural function. It is through sensory integration that the many parts of the nervous system work together so that a person can interact with the environment effectively.

**Stability:** The ability to maintain or regain equilibrium. It is a dynamic process underlying postural control and controlled movement.

**Standard Swallow:** The action of the tongue that is characterized by lip closure, tongue-tip elevation and a controlled movement of the bolus, liquid or saliva back over the tongue to effect a safe swallow.

**Strength:** For our purposes, strength is the force necessary to sustain a movement in rapid sequence. Strength is a component in the development of speech clarity. Strength in the oral articulators can be improved through repetition, during therapeutic feeding, oral placement and by direct work on isolated speech sound movements.

**Superimposed Stability:** Using an outside force to create stability in the body or in isolated muscle groups to facilitate mobility in higher level muscle movements for improved function.

**Supine:** Lying with the face upwards.

**Symmetry:** Equal balance of structure, skill levels, or movement. Equal movement in corresponding extremities or muscle groups on opposite sides of the body.

**Tactile Cue:** When touch to the mouth is used to supply information.

**Tactile Defensiveness:** A learned pattern of negative behavior in response to sensory input. This behavior is learned secondary to sensory deficits: hyposensitivity, hypersensitivity, mixed sensitivity or fluctuating sensitivity. The behavioral component must be addressed by developing trust, prior to or in conjunction with working on normalizing the sensory system.

**Target Placement:** The standard placement of the oral articulators in response to the introduction of a therapy tool or through verbal instruction.

**Targeted Speech Sound:** The phoneme that you have chosen to have your client work on at the level of production after you have completed the prerequisite hierarchy of: (1) awareness, (2) placement and (3) adequate strength/muscle memory.

**Therapeutic Horn Blowing:** A therapeutic approach, developed by Sara Rosenfeld-Johnson, which uses a hierarchy of horns to work on improving abdominal grading, controlled oral airflow, velopharyngeal functioning, saliva control and ultimately developing speech clarity.

**Therapeutic Straw Drinking:** A therapeutic approach, developed by Sara Rosenfeld-Johnson, which uses a hierarchy of straws to address the goals of improving tongue retraction/grading, lip rounding, feeding skills, and the development of standard speech sound production.

**Tongue Grading Hierarchy:** Refer to the Eight Levels of Tongue Grading.

**Traditional Therapy:** Speech therapy which stresses auditory stimulation in addition to visual stimulation to correct speech clarity errors.

**True Lateralization:** When the back of the tongue retracts and stabilizes as the tongue-tip touches the inside of the lower back molar on alternating sides of the mouth, without associated jaw movements.

213

**Velopharyngeal Closure:** When the back of the velum and the pharyngeal wall make contact, thereby inhibiting air from escaping through the nose.

**Velopharyngeal Function:** When the velum makes contact with the pharyngeal wall for oral directionality of airflow and then moves away from the pharyngeal wall for nasal directionality of airflow.

**Verbal Cue:** When a single word, phrase, or sentence is used to supply information.

**Visual Cue:** When an object, picture, or written word is used to supply information.

**Voicing Errors:** Phoneme errors which are secondary to confusion in timing; the vocal folds vibrate when they are not supposed to or they do not vibrate when they should.

**Volume:** Loudness.

# References:

**Adams, S.G.** 1997. Hypokinetic dysarthria in Parkinson's disease. In *Clinical Management of Sensorimotor Speech Disorders.* ed. M. R. McNeal, 261-285. New York: Thieme Medical Publishers.

**Alba, J., Quest** Engineering Report. 2007. Test Report # Q08024. *Horns and Straws in a Hierarchy of Difficulty.* Billerica, MA.

**Alexander, R. 1987**. Oral-motor treatment for infants and young children with cerebral palsy. *Seminars in Speech and Language.* 8 (1): 87-100.

**Alexander, R.** 1990. *Oral-motor and respiratory-phonatory assessment. In Interdisciplinary Assessment of Infants: A Guide for Early Intervention Professionals.* ed. E.D. Gibbs and D.M. Teti, 63-74. Baltimore: Paul H. Brookes.

**American Psychological Association.** 1994. Publication manual of the American Psychological Association. 4th ed. Washington, DC. American Psychological Association.

**American Speech-Language-Hearing Association.** 1991. The role of the speech-language pathologist in management of oral myofunctional disorders. ASHA 33: Suppl. 5. 7.

**American Speech-Language-Hearing Association.** 1993. Orofacial myofunctional disorders: knowledge and skills. ASHA 35: Suppl.10. 21-23.

**Amerman, D., R. Daniloff, and K. Moll.** 1970. Lip and jaw coarticulation. *Speech Hearing Research* 13:147-161.

**Armstrong, L.** 2006. *ACSM's Guidelines for Exercise Testing and Prescription.* 7th ed. Baltimore, MD: Lippincott Williams & Wilkins.

**Arvedson, J.C., and L. Brodsky. eds.** 1993. *Pediatric Swallowing and Feeding Assessment and Management.* 249-291. San Diego: Singular Publishing Group.

**ASHA.** 1990. Issues in oral motor, feeding, swallowing, and respiratory phonatory assessment and intervention. A Building Blocks Module.

**ASHA.** 2007. Childhood apraxia of speech. Technical report.

**Ayres, A.J.** 1972b. *Sensory Integration and Learning Disorders.* Los Angeles: Western Psychological Services.

**Ayres, A.J.** 1976. *The Effect of Sensory Integrative Therapy on Learning Disabled Children: The Final Report of a Research Project.* Los Angeles: University of Southern California.

**Ayres, A.J.** 1979. *Sensory Integration and the Child.* Los Angeles: Western Psychological Services.

**Bahr, D. C.** 2000. *Oral-motor Assessment and Treatment.* Needham, MA: Allyn and Bacon.

**Bahr, D. C.** 2001. *Oral Motor Assessment and Treatment: Ages and Stages.* Boston: Allyn and Bacon.

**Bahr, D.** 2008. A topical bibliography on oral motor assessment and treatment. *Oral Motor Institute* 2 (1). Available from www.oralmotorinstitute.org.

**Baker, E.,** and S. McLeod. 2004. Evidence-based management of phonological impairment in children. *Child Language Teaching and Therapy* 20 (3): 261-285.

**Barnes, J.F.** 1990. Myofascial Release: *A Comprehensive Evaluatory and Treatment Approach*. John F. Barnes, PT and Rehabilitation Services. Paoli, PA.

**Bartlett, D.** 1997. Primitive reflexes and early motor development. Journal of Development and Behavioral Pediatrics 18:143-150.

**Bauman-Waengler, J.** 2008. *Articulatory and Phonological Impairments*. Pearson.

**Beidler, L.M.,** and R. L. Smallman. 1965. Renewal of cells within taste buds. *Journal of Cellular Biology* 27 (2): 265-272.

**Berntha l, John,** and N. W. Bankson. 1998. *Articulation and Phonological Disorders*. 299-369. Allyn and Bacon.

**Berry, M. F.** 1969. *Language Disorders of Children*. New York: Appleton-Century-Crofts.

**Beukelman, D.R.,** and P. Mirenda. 1992. *Augmentative and Alternative Communication: Management of Severe Communication Disorders in Children and Adults*. 230. Baltimore: Paul H. Brookes.

**Bly, L.** 1983. *The Components of Normal Movement During the First Year of Life and Abnormal Motor Development*. Chicago: Neuro-Developmental Treatment Association.

**Bobath, B.** 1970. *Adult Hemiplegia Evaluation and Treatment*. London: William Heinemann Medical Books.

**Bobath, B.** 1971. Motor development, its effect on general development, and application to the treatment of cerebral palsy. *Physiotherapy* 57 (11): 526-532.

**Bobath, K.** 1971. The normal postural reflex mechanism and its deviation in children with cerebral palsy. *Physiotherapy* 57 (11): 515-525.

**Boehme, R.** 1990. *The Hypotonic Child: Treatment for Postural Control, Endurance, Strength, and Sensory Organization*. Tucson, AZ: Therapy Skill Builders.

**Braun, M. A.,** and M. M. Palmer. 1986. A pilot study of oral-motor dysfunction in "at-risk" infants. *Physical & Occupational Therapy in Pediatrics* 5 (4): 13-25.

**Brooks, V. B.** 1986. *The Neural Basis of Motor Control*. New York: Oxford University Press.

**Brookshire, R. H.** 1997. *An Introduction to Neurogenic Communication Disorders*. 5th ed. Saint Louis: Mosby Year Book.

**Brown, J. R., F. L. Darley,** and A. E. Aronson. 1970. Ataxic dysarthria. *International Journal of Neurology* 7:302-318.

**Burpee, J. D.** 1999. "Sensory Integration, Applied Behavior Analysis, and Floor Time." Baltimore: Care Resources, Inc. (workshop).

**Cameol, S. O., S. M. Marks,** and L. Weik. 1999. The speech-language pathologist: Key role in the diagnosis of Velocardiofacial syndrome. *American Journal of Speech-Language Pathology* B: 23-32.

**Cannito, M. P.,** and T. P. Marquardt. 1997. *Ataxic Dysarthria. In Clinical Management of Sensorimotor Speech Disorders*. ed. M. R. 217-247. New York: Thieme Medical Publishers.

**Caruso, A. J., and E. A. Strand.** 1999. Motor speech disorders in children: Definitions, background, and a theoretical framework. In Clinical Management of Motor Speech Disorders in Children. ed. A. J. Caruso and E. A. Strand. 1-27. New York: Thieme Medical Publishers.

**Chertkow, H., and D. Bub.** 1994. Functional activation and cognition: The 0-15 PET subtraction method. In *Localization and Neuroimaging in Neuropsychology*. ed. A. Kertesz. 152-184. San Diego: Academic Press.

**Christensen, M., and M. Hanson.** 1981. An investigation of the efficacy of oral-motor therapy as a precursor to articulation therapy for pre-first grade children. *Journal of Speech and Hearing Disorders* 46. Dewey 1993.

**Clark, H. M.** 2003. Neuromuscular treatments for speech and swallowing. *American Journal of Speech Language Pathology* 12:400-415.

**Clark, H. M.** 2005. *Clinical decision making and oral motor treatments.* The ASHA Leader. 8-9, 34-35. http://www.asha.org/about/publications/leader-online/ archives/2005/f050614b.htm.

**Crary, M. A.** 1993. *Developmental Motor Speech Disorders*. San Diego: Singular Publishing Group.

**Darley, F., A. E. Aronson, and J. R. Brown.** 1975. Motor Speech Disorders. Philadelphia: W. B. Sauders.

**DeMyer, W. E.** 1994. *Technique of the Neurologic Examination: A Programmed Text*. 4th ed. New York: McGraw-Hill. Health Professions Division.

**Densem, J. F., G. A. Nuthall, J. Bushnell, and J. Horn.** 1989. Effectiveness of a sensory integrative therapy program for children with perceptual-motor deficits. *Journal of Learning Disabilities* 22:221-229.

**Duffy, J. R.** 1995. *Motor Speech Disorders: Substrates, Differential Diagnosis and Management*. St. Louis: Mosby Year Book.

**Dworkin, J. P., and R. A. Culatta.** 1996. *The Dworkin-Culatta Oral Mechanism Examination and Treatment System*. Nicholasville, KY. Edgewood Press.

**Feldenkrais, M.** 1972. *Awareness Through Movement: Health Exercise for Personal Growth*. New York: Harper & Row.

**Feldenkrais, M.** 1975. *Awareness through Movement. The 1975 Annual Handbook for Group Facilitators*. San Francisco: University Associates Publishers.

**Field, T.** 1995. Massage therapy for infants and children. *Journal of Developmental Behavioral Pediatrics* 16 (2): 105-111.

**Field, T.** 1998. Massage therapy effects. *American Psychology* 53 (12): 1270-1281.

**Fisher, A.G., E. A. Murray, and A. C. Bundy. eds**. 1991. *Sensory Integration: Theory and Practice*. Philadelphia: F.A. Davis.

**Fisher, A. G.** 1991. Vestibular-proprioceptive processing and bilateral integration and sequencing deficits. In *Sensory integration: Theory and Practice*. ed. A.G. Fisher, E. A. Murray, and A. C. Bundy. 71-107. Philadelphia: F. A. Davis.

**Fisher, A. G., and E. A. Murray.** 1991. Introduction to sensory integration theory. In *Sensory Integration: Theory and Practice*. ed. A. G. Fisher, E. A. Murray, and A. C. Bundy. 1-26. Philadelphia: F. A. Davis.

**Fletcher, S., R. Casteel, and D. Bradley.** 1961. Tongue thrust swallow, speech articulation, and age. *Journal of Speech and Hearing Disorders* 26:219-225.

**Fletcher, S.** 1974. *Tongue Thrust in Swallowing and Speaking*. Austin, TX: Learning Concepts.

**Fletcher, S.G**. 1992. *Articulation: A Physiological Approach*. San Diego, CA: Singular.

**Geschwind, N.** 1965. Disconnexion syndromes in animals and man. *Brain* 88: 237-294, 585-644.

**Gierut, J.** 1998. Treatment efficacy: Functional phonological disorders in children. *Journal of Speech, Language, and Hearing Research* 41:S85-S101.

**Glennen, S. L., and D. C. DeCoste.** 1997. *Handbook of Augmentative and Alternative Communication*. San Diego: Singular Publishing Group.

**Goldman-Eisler, F.** 1968. *Psycholinguistics: Experiments in Spontaneous Speech*. New York: Academic Press.

**Green, J. R., C. A. Moore, J. L. Ruark, P. R. Rodda, W. T. Morvee, and M. J. VanWitzenburg.** 1997. Development of chewing in children from 12 to 48 months: Longitudinal study of EMG patterns. *Journal of Neurophysiology* 77:2704-2716.

**Greenspan, S. I.** 1995. *The Challenging Child: Understanding, Raising, and Enjoying the Five "Difficult" Types of Children*. Reading, MA: Addison-Wesley.

**Greenspan, S. I.** 1997. *The Growth of the Mind and the Endangered Origins of Intelligence*. Reading, MA: Addison-Wesley.

**Greenspan, S. I., and S. Wieder.** 1998. The Child with Special Needs: Encouraging Intellectual and Emotional growth. 232. Reading, MA: Perseus Books.

**Groher, M. E. ed.** 1997. *Dysphagia: Diagnosis and Management*. 3rd ed. Boston: Butterworth-Heinemann Medical.

**Hammer, D.** 2007. "Childhood Apraxia of Speech: New Perspectives on Assessment and Treatment." Las Vegas, NV: The Childhood Apraxia of Speech Association. (workshop).

**Hanson, M., and M. Cohen.** 1973. Effects of form and function on swallowing and the developing dentition. *American Journal of Orthodontics* 64:63-82.

**Hawk, S., and E. H. Young.** 1938. *Moto-Kinesthetic Speech Training*. Stanford: Stanford University Press.

**Hayden, D. A., and P. A. Square.** 1999. *Verbal Motor Production Assessment for Children*. San Antonio, TX: Psychological Corporation.

**Heitler, S** 1993. *David Decides About Thumb Sucking*. Denver, CO Reading Matters.

**Hickman, L. A.** 1997. *The Apraxia Profile*. San Antonio, TX: Communication Skill Builders.

**Hodge, M. M.** 2002. Nonspeech oral motor treatment approaches for dysarthria: Perspectives on controversial clinical practices. *Perspectives in Neurophysiology and Neurogenic Speech Disorders* 12 (4): 22-28.

**Howard, D., K. Patterson, R. Wise, W. D. Brown, K Friston, C. Weiller, and R. Frackowiak.** 1992. The cortical localization of the lexicons. *Brain* 115:1769-1782.

**Illingworth, R. S., and J. Lister.** 1964. The critical or sensitive period, with special reference to certain feeding problems in infants and children. *The Journal of Pediatrics* 65 (6): 839-848.

**Jelm, J. M.** 1990. *Oral-Motor/Feeding Rating Scale*. Tucson, AZ: Therapy Skill Builders.

**Jordan, L., J. Hardy, and H. Morris.** 1978. Performance of children with good and poor articulation on tasks of tongue placement. *Journal of Speech and Hearing Research* 21:429-439.

**Kabat, H., and M. Knott.** 1948. Principles of neuromuscular re-education. *Physical Therapy Review* 28:107-110.

**Kaufman, N. R.** 1995. *The Kaufman Speech Praxis Test for Children*. Detroit, MI: Wayne State University Press.

**Kent, R** 1994. *Reference Manual for Communication Sciences and Disorders*. Pro-Ed Inc.

**Kent, R. D.** 1999. *Motor control: Neurophysiology and functional development. In Clinical Management of Motor Speech Disorders in Children*. ed. A. J. Caruso and E. A. Strand. 29-71. New York: Thieme Medical Publishers.

**Kent, R. D.** July 2008. Theory in the balance. *Perspectives on Speech Science and Orofacial Disorders* 18:15-21.

**Klein, M. D., and S. E. Morris.** 1999. *Mealtime Participation Guide*. San Antonio, TX: Therapy Skill Builders.

**Knott, M., and D. E. Voss.** 1956. *Proprioceptive Neuromuscular Facilitation: Patterns and Techniques*. New York: Harper & Row.

**Koomar, J. A., and A. C. Bundy.** 1991. The art and science of creating direct intervention from theory. *In Sensory Integration: Theory and Practice*. ed. A. Murray, A. C. Bundy, E. A. Murray, and A. G. Fisher. 251-314. Philadelphia: F. A. Davis.

**Kranowitz, C. S.** 1998. *The Out-of-Sync Child: Recognizing and Coping with Sensory Integration Dysfunction*. New York: Berkley Publishing Group.

**Kuhn, C. M., S. M. Schanberg, T. Field, R. Symanski, E. Zimmerman, F. Scafidi, and J. Roberts.** 1991. Tactile-kinesthetic stimulation effects on sympathetic and adrenocortical function in preterm infants. *Journal of Pediatrics* 119 (3): 434-440.

**Kumin, L.** 1997. "Oral Motor Assessment and Treatment in Infants, Children, and Adolescents with Down syndrome." Columbia, MD. (workshop).

**Kumin, L., and D. C. Bahr.** 1997. "Oral Motor Skills: Assessment and Intervention for Infants, Toddlers, Children, and Adolescents with Down syndrome." Baltimore: Loyola College. (workshop).

**Kumin, L., and D. C. Bahr.** 1999. Patterns of feeding, eating, and drinking in young children with Down syndrome with oral motor concerns. *Down Syndrome Quarterly* 4 (2): 1-8.

**Kumin, L., M. Goodman, and C. Councill.** 1996. Comprehensive speech and language intervention for school-aged children with Down syndrome. *Down Syndrome Quarterly* 1 (1): 1-17.

**Langley, M. B., and C. Thomas, C.** 1991. Introduction to the neurodevelopmental approach. In *Neurodevelopmental Strategies for Managing Communication Disorders in Children with Severe Motor Dysfunction*. 1-28. ed. M. B. Langley and L. J. Lombardino. Austin, TX: Pro-Ed.

**Lass, Norman J. and Raymond Kent.** 1996. *Principles of Experimental Phonetics*. Mosby. 3-45.

**Levitt, Sofie.** 1975. *Treatment of Cerebral Palsy and Motor Delay*. Blackwell Scientific Publications.

**Liberman, S. M.** 1957. Some results of research on speech perception. *Journal of the Acoustical Society of America* 29:117-123.

**Logemann, J. A.** 1992. "Diagnostic Related Swallowing Disorders and Their Management (Course II)." Detroit, MI: Northern Speech Services. (workshop).

**Logemann, J. A.** 1997. *Evaluation and Treatment of Swallowing Disorders*. 2nd ed. Austin, TX: Pro- Ed.

**Long, A. D., D. C. Bahr, and L. Kumin.** 1998. "The Battery for Oral-motor Behavior in Children." Baltimore: Loyola College in Maryland. (unpublished test)

**Love, R. J., E. L. Hagerman, and E. G. Tiami.** 1980. Speech performance, dysphasia and oral reflexes in cerebral palsy. *Journal of Speech and Hearing Disorders* 45:59-75.

**Love, R. J., and W. G. Webb.** 1996. *Neurology for the Speech-Language Pathologist*. 3rd ed. Boston: Butterworth -Heinemann.

**Maas, E., D. A. Robin, S. N. Austermann Hula, S. E. Freedman, G. Wulf, K. J. Ballard, and R. A. Schmidt.** 2008. Principles of motor learning in treatment of motor speech disorders. *American Journal of Speech-Language Pathology* 17:277-298.

**Macaluso-Haynes, S.** 1978. Developmental apraxia of speech: Symptoms and treatment. In *Clinical Management of Neurogenic Communication Disorders*. ed. D. F. Johns. 243-250. Boston: Little, Brown.

**Marshalla, P.** 2004. *Oral-Motor Techniques in Articulation and Phonological Therapy*. Mill Creek, WA: Marshalla Speech and Language.

**Mason, R., and W. Proffit,** 1974. The tongue thrust controversy: background and recommendations. *Journal of Speech and Hearing Disorders* 39:115-132.

**Matthews, P. B. C.** 1988. Proprioceptors and their contribution to somatosensory mapping: Complex messages require complex processing. *Canadian Journal of Physiology and Pharmacology* 66:430-438.

**McClure, V. S.** 1989. *Infant massage: A handbook for Loving Parents.* rev. ed. New York: Bantam Books.

**McDonald, E. T.** 1964. *Articulation Testing and Treatment: .4 Sensory-Motor Approach*. Pittsburgh: Stanwix.

**McNeil, M. R., D. A. Robin, and R. A. Schmidt.** 1997. Apraxia of speech: Definition, differentiation, and treatment. In *Clinical Management of Sensorimotor Speech Disorders*. 311-344. ed. M. R. McNeil. New York: Thieme Medical Publishers.

**Melzack, R., K. W. Konrad, and B. Dubrovsky.** 1969. Prolonged changes in central nervous system activity produced by somatic and reticular stimulation. *Experimental Neurology* 25: 416-428.

**Meyer, T.** 1984. *Help Your Baby Build a Healthy Body: A New Exercise and Massage Program for the First Five Formative Years.* New York: Crown Publishers.

**Michi, K., Y. Yamashita, S. Imai, and N. Suzuli.** 1993. Role of visual feedback treatment for defective /s/ sounds in patients with cleft palate. *Journal of Speech and Hearing Research* 36:277-285

**Miller, J. F., and M. Leddy.** 1998. Down syndrome, the impact of speech production on language development. In *Exploring the Speech-Language Connection.* 163-177, 234. ed. R. Paul. Baltimore: Paul H. Brookes.

**Mohr, J. D.** 1990. Management of the trunk in adult hemiplegia: The Bobath concept. *Topics in Neurology* Lesson 1: 1-11.

**Montagu, A.** 1986. *Touching: The Human Significance of the Skin.* 3rd ed. New York: Harper & Row.

**Moore, C., and J. Ruark.** 1996. Does speech emerge from earlier appearing oral motor behaviors? *Journal of Speech and Hearing Research* 39:1034-1047.

**Morris, S. E.** 1982. *The Normal Acquisition of Oral Feeding Skills: Implications for Assessment and Treatment.* Santa Barbara, CA: Therapeutic Media.

**Morris, S. E.** 1985. Developmental implications for the management of feeding problems in neurologically impaired infants. *Seminars in Speech and Language* 6 (4): 293-315.

**Morris, S. E.** 1989. Development of oral-motor skills in the neurologically impaired child receiving non-oral feedings. *Dysphagia* 3 (3): 135-154.

**Morris, S. E., and M.D. Klein.** 1987. *Pre-feeding skills: A Comprehensive Resource for Feeding Development.* 2d ed. San Antonio, TX: Therapy Skill Builders.

**Morris, S. E., and M. D. Klein.** 2000. *Pre-feeding Skills: A Comprehensive Resource for Mealtime Development.* 2nd ed. San Antonio, TX: Therapy Skill Builders.

**Murdoch, B. E., E. C. Thompson, and D. G. Theodoros.** 1997. Spastic dysarthria. In *Clinical Management of Sensorimotor Speech Disorders.* 287-310. ed. M. R. McNeil. New York: Thieme Medical Publishers.

**Mysak, E.** 1983. Treatment of deviant phonological systems: Cerebral palsy. In *Dysarthria and Apraxia: Current Therapy of Communication Disorders.* 3-23. ed. W.H. Perkins. New York: Thieme-Stratton Inc.

**Nelson, C. A., and R. M. de Benabib.** 1991. Sensory preparation of the oral-motor area. In *Neurodevelopmental Strategies for Managing Communication Disorders in Children with Severe Motor Dysfunction.* 131-158. ed. M. B. Langley and L. J. Lombardino. Austin, TX: Pro-Ed.

**Nelson, C. A., M. M. Meek, and J. C. Moore.** 1994. *Head-neck Treatment Issues as a Base for Oral Motor Function.* Albuquerque, NM: Clinician's View.

**Nicolosi, L., E. Harryman, and J. Kresheck.** 1989. *Terminology of Communication Disorders: Speech-Language-Hearing.* 3rd ed. Baltimore: Williams & Wilkins.

**Oetter, P., E. W. Richter, and S. M. Frick.** 1995. M.O.R.E.: *Integrating the Mouth with Sensory and Postural Functions.* 2d ed. Hugo, MN: PDP Press.

**Ong, D., and M. Stone.** 1998. Three-dimensional vocal tract shapes in /r/ and /l/: A study of MRI, ultrasound, electropalatography, and acoustics. *Phonoscope* 1: 1-13.

**Overland, L.** 1999. *Feeding Therapy: A Hands-On Experience.* Tucson, AZ: Innovative Therapists International." (video).

**Palmer, J. M.** 1993. *Anatomy for Speech and Hearing.* 4th ed. Baltimore: Williams & Wilkins.

**Palmer, P., D. Jaffe, T. McCulloch, E. Finnegan, D. Van Daele, and E. Luschei.** 2008. Quantitative contributions of the muscles of the tongue, floor-of-mouth, jaw, and velum to tongue-to-palate pressure generation. *Journal of Speech, Language and Hearing Research* 51:828-835.

**Perkell, J. S., F. H. Guenther, H. Lane, M. L. Matthies, P. Perrier, and J. Vick, et al.** 2000. A theory of speech motor control and supporting data from speakers with normal hearing and with profound hearing loss. *Journal of Phonetics* 28 (3): 233-272.

**Perkell, J. S., H. Guenther, H. Lane, M. L. Matthies, R. Wilhelms-Tricarico, and J. Wozniak, et al**. 1997. Speech motor control: Acoustic goals, saturation effects, auditory feedback and internal models. *Speech Communication* 22 (2-3): 227-250.

**Pierce, R. B.** 1978. Tongue Thrust: *A Look at Oral Myofunctional Disorders.* Lincoln, NE: Cliffs-Notes.

**Pierce, R. B.** 1993. *Swallow Right: An Exercise Program to Correct Swallowing Patterns.* Tucson, AZ: Communication Skill Builders.

**Powell, T.W.** 2008. An integrated evaluation of nonspeech oral motor treatments. *Language, Speech, and Hearing Services in the Schools* 39:422-427.

**Redstone, F.** 1991. Respiratory components of communication. In *Neurodevelopmental Strategies for Managing Communication Disorders in Children with Severe Motor Dysfunction.* ed. M. B. Langley, and L. J. Lombardino. 29-48. Austin, TX: Pro-Ed.

**Ringel, R. L., and S.J. Ewanowski.** 1965. Oral perception I. Two-point discrimination. *Journal of Speech and Hearing Research* 8 (4): 235, 389-398.

**Ringel, R. L., and H. M. Fletcher.** 1967. Oral perception III. Texture discrimination. *Journal of Speech and Hearing Research* 10 (3): 642-649.

**Rood, M. S.** 1954. Neurophysiological reactions as a basis for physical therapy. *Physical Therapy Review* 34:444-449.

**Rosenbek, J. C., and Associates.** 1973. A treatment for apraxia of speech in adults. *Journal of Speech and Hearing Disorders* 38:462-472.

**Rosenbek, J. C., and L. L. LaPointe.** 1978. The dysarthrias: Description, diagnosis, and treatment. In *Clinical Management of Neurogenic Communicative Disorders.* ed. D. F. Johns. 251-310. Boston: Little, Brown.

**Rosenfeld-Johnson, S.** 1997. The oral-motor myths of Down syndrome. Advance.

**Rosenfeld-Johnson, S.** 1999. *Oral-Motor Exercises for Speech Clarity.* Tucson, AZ: Innovative Therapists International.

**Rosenfeld-Johnson, S.** 1999. *A Three-Part Treatment Plan for Oral-Motor Therapy*. Tucson, AZ: Innovative Therapists International (video).

**Rosenfeld-Johnson, S.** 1999. Straws as therapy tools. *Advance*.

**Rosenfeld-Johnson, S.** 2001. Effective exercises for a short frenum. *Advance*.

**Rosenfeld-Johnson, S.** 2001. *Oral-Motor Exercises for Speech Clarity*. Tucson, AZ: Innovative Therapists International.

**Rosenfeld-Johnson, S.** 2004. *Oral-Motor Exercises for Speech Clarity.* 26th World Congress of the International Association of Logopedics and Phoniatrics. Brisbane, Australia.

**Rosenfeld-Johnson, S.** 2005. *Assessment and Treatment of the Jaw- Putting It All Together: Sensory, Feeding and Speech*. Tucson, AZ: Innovative Therapists International.

**Rosenfeld-Johnson, S.** 2005. *Assessment and Treatment of the Jaw*. DVD Tucson, AZ: Innovative Therapists International.

**Rosenfeld-Johnson, S.** 2009. *Oral Placement Therapy for /s/ and /z/.* Tucson, AZ: Innovative Therapists International.

**Rosenfeld-Johnson, S., and J. Gray.** 2008. The role of the jaw for feeding and speech. *Advance* 18 (35).

**Rosenfeld-Johnson, S., and J. Gray.** 2008. Strategies to eliminate maladaptive oral habits. *Advance for Speech-Language Pathologists & Audiologists Online*, Speech and Hearing Resource Center: Speech and Voice Disorders. Accessed online at www.advanceweb.com/speech.

**Roth, Froma P., and Colleen K. Worthington.** 1997. *Treatment Resource Manual for Speech-Language Pathology*. 114. Singular Publishing Group, Inc. Dept. Hearing and Speech Sciences. University of Maryland.

**Royeen, C. B., & Lane, S. J.** 1991. Tactile processing and sensory defensiveness. In *Sensory Integration: Theory and Practice*. 108-133. ed. A. G. Fisher, E. A. Murray, & A. C. Bundy. Philadelphia: F. A. Davis.

**Ruark, J. L., & Moore, C. A.** 1997. Coordination of lip muscle activity by two-year-old children during speech and nonspeech tasks. *Journal of Speech, Language, and Hearing Research* 40:1373-1385.

**Ruscello, D. M.** 2008. Nonspeech oral motor treatment issues related to children with developmental speech sound disorders. *Language, Speech, and Hearing Services in the Schools* 39:380-391.

**Savrson, R. H.** 1961. *Motor Phonetics*. Amsterdam, Netherlands: North Holland.

**Scherzer, A., and I. Tscharnuter.** 1982. *Early Diagnosis and Therapy in Cerebral Palsy*. New York: Marcel Dekker.

**Schmidt, R. A.** 1975. A schema theory of discrete motor skill learning. *Psychological Review* 82:225-260.

**Schmidt, R. A.** 1988. *Motor Control and Learning: A Behavioral Emphasis*. 2nd ed. Champaign, IL: Human Kinetics.

**Schmidt, R. A.** 2003. Motor schema theory after 27 years: Reflections and implications for a new theory. *Research Quarterly for Exercise and Sport* 74:366-375.

**Secord, W., S. Boyce, J. Donohur, R. Fox, and R. Shine.** 2007. *Eliciting Sounds: Techniques and Strategies for Clinicians.* Cengage Learning.

**Sherrington, C. S.** 1913. Reflex inhibition as a factor in the co-ordination of movements and postures. *Quarterly Journal of Experimental Physiology* 6:251.

**Shipley, K. G., J. G. McMee.** 1992. *Assessment in Speech-Language Pathology: A Resource Manual.* San Diego: Singular Publishing Group.

**Sieg, K. W., and S. P. Adams.** 1985. *Illustrated Essentials of Musculoskeletal Anatomy.* Gainesville, FL: Megabooks.

**Smith, A., C. M. Weber, J. Newton, and M. Denny.** 1991. Developmental and age-related changes in reflexes of the human jaw-closing system. *Electroencephalography and Clinical Neurophysiology* 81:118-128.

**Stilwell, J. M., T.K. Crowe, and L. W. McCallum.** 1978. Postrotary nystagmus duration as a function of communication disorders. *American Journal of Occupational Therapy* 32:222-228.

***Stone, M., and A. Lundberg.*** 1998. Three-dimensional tongue surface shapes of English consonants and vowels. In *Neuromotor Speech Disorders: Nature, Assessment, and Management.* 3-25. ed. M. P. Cannito, K. M. Yorkston, and D. R. Beukelman. Baltimore: Paul H. Brookes.

**Strand, E., and M. Sullivan.** 2001. Evidence-based practice guidelines for dysarthria: Management for Velopharyngeal function. *Journal of Medical Speech-Language Pathology* 9:257-274.

**Stray-Gundersen, K. ed.** 1995. *Babies with Down Syndrome: A New Parents' Guide.* 2nd ed. 236. Bethesda, MD: Woodbine House.

**Sullivan, P. E., P. D. Markos, and M. D. Minor.** 1982. *An Integrated Approach to Therapeutic Exercise: Theory and Clinical Application.* Reston, VA: Reston Publishing.

**Tuchman, D. N., and R. S. Walter. eds.** 1994. *Disorders of Feeding and Swallowing in Infants and Children: Pathophysiology, Diagnosis and Treatment.* San Diego: Singular Publishing Group.

**Walter, R. S.** 1994. Issues surrounding the development of feeding and swallowing. In *Disorders of Feeding and Swallowing in Infants and Children: Pathophysiology, Diagnosis and Treatment.* 27-35. ed. D. N. Tuchman and R. S. Walter. San Diego: Singular Publishing Group.

**Weisz, S.** 1938. Studies in equilibrium reactions. *Journal of Nervous and Mental Disease* 88:150-162.

**Wertz, R. T.** 1978. Neuropathologies of speech and language: An introduction to patient management. In *Clinical Management of Neurogenic Communicative Disorders.* 1-101. ed. D. F. Johns. Boston: Little, Brown.

**Wertz, R. T., L. L. LaPointe, and J. C. Rosenbek.** 1991. *Apraxia of Speech in Adults: The Disorder and its Management.* San Diego: Singular Publishing Group.

**Westermann, G., and E. R. Miranda.** 2004. A new model of sensorimotor coupling in the development of speech. *Brain and Language* 89:393-400.

**Wheeler, L., C. J. Burke, and R. M. Reitan.** 1963. An application of discriminant functions to the problem of predicting brain damage using behavioral variables. *Perceptual and Motor Skills* 16:417-440.

**White, B. L.** 1995. *The First Three Years of Life*. rev. ed. New York: Prentice-Hall.

**Wilbarger, P., and J. L. Wilbarger.** 1991. Sensory Defensiveness in Children Aged 2-12: *An Intervention Guide for Parents and Other Caregivers*. Santa Barbara, CA: Avanti Educational Programs.

**Wilson, E. M., J. R. Green, Y. Yunusova, and C. A. Moore.** 2008. Task specificity in early oral motor development. *Seminars in Speech and Language* 29:257-266.

**Winders, P. C.** 1997. *Topics in Down Syndrome: Gross Motor Skills in Children with Down Syndrome: A Guide for Parents and Professionals*. Bethesda, MD: Woodbine House.

**Yarrom, R., U. Sagher, Y. Havivi, I. J. Peled, and M. R. Wexler.** 1986. Myofibers in tongues of Down syndrome. *Journal of Neurological Science* 73:279-287.

**Young, E. H., and S. S. Hawk.** 1955. *Moto-Kinesthestic Speech Training*. Stanford, CA: Stanford University Press.

**Zemlin, W. R.** 1998. *Speech and Hearing Science: Anatomy and Physiology*. 4th ed. Boston: Allyn and Bacon.

**Ziev, M. S. R.** 1999. Earliest intervention: Speech-language pathology services in the neonatal intensive care unit. ASHA. 32-36.

**Zraick, R. I., and L. L LaPointe.** 1997. Hyperkinetic dysarthria. In *Clinical Management of Sensorimotor Speech Disorders*. 237, 249-260. ed. M. R. McNeil. New York: Thieme Medical Publishers.

**Forthcoming Titles by Sara Rosenfeld-Johnson:**

*Oral Placement Therapy (OPT) for Voice Disorders*

*Oral Placement Therapy (OPT) for /n/, /t/, /d/ and /l/*

**Other Titles by Sara Rosenfeld-Johnson available from TalkTools:**

**Books and Programs:**

*Assessment and Treatment of the Jaw: - Putting It All Together: Sensory, Feeding and Speech*

*HOMEWORK Book* (with Susan Money)

*Oral Placement Therapy (OPT) for /s/ and /z/*

*Drooling Remediation Program*

*The Ice Stick Program* (with Renee Roy Hill)

*Sensory Stix Program* (with Robyn Merkel)

**DVDS - Continuing Education- ASHA and AOTA Approved:**

*A Three-Part Treatment Plan for Oral-Motor Therapy*

*Assessment and Treatment of the Jaw: Sensory, Feeding and Speech*

*Horns as Therapy Tools*

*Straws as Therapy Tools*

*Bubbles as Therapy Tool*

*Diagnosis and Program Planning*

*As A Parent What Can I Do?* (not approved for CEUs)